Live Food

JUICES

For
Vim ...
Vigor ...
Vitality ...
Long Life ...

by

H. E. Kirschner, M. D.

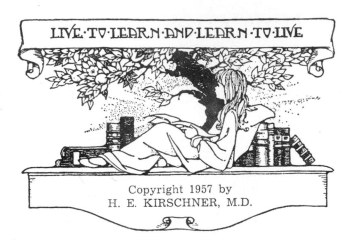

LIVE·TO·LEARN·AND·LEARN·TO·LIVE

First Printing, January, 1957
Second Printing, May, 1957
Third Printing, April, 1958
Fourth Printing, October, 1958
Fifth Printing, February, 1959
Sixth Printing, July, 1959
Seventh Printing, December, 1959
Eighth Printing, June, 1960
Ninth Printing, December, 1960
Tenth Printing, June, 1961
Eleventh Printing, June, 1963
Twelfth Printing, February, 1964
Thirteenth Printing, November, 1964
Fourteenth Printing, August, 1965

Published and Distributed by

H. E. KIRSCHNER PUBLICATIONS

P.O. Box 361

Monrovia, California

PRICE $2.00

PRINTED
IN
U.S.A.

Introduction . . .

EACH one of us in this life has had a different set of experiences and so we should, as much as possible, profit by the experiences of others if we are smart. You might say that we are the sum of our experiences, the people we have met, the places we have been, the books we have read, etc. ad infinitum. So it is difficult at times to be broad minded enough to listen to other people's experiences, especially when they differ so much from our own pet ideas, habits, customs. Some one once said: "People are always down on things they are not up on." How true — how foolish, too. If "experience is the best teacher" why not listen to the experiences of Dr. Kirschner, who has practiced his profession for over fifty years, very successfully, in a way that is quite different from the average general practitioner. This could be fascinating, perhaps frustrating at first, but I assure you a rewarding experience.

So long as we look at disease as being due to the presence of something, a germ, a toxin, a virus, we can not conceive that disease may be due to the absence of something, and yet more and more medical men are becoming aware of what we call deficiency diseases, the accepted ones being beri beri, rickets, pellegra and scurvy. If these diseased states are due to deficiencies of certain protective food factors (or vitamins), why not many other diseased states and syndromes. Just so long as we look for specific drugs to cure specific diseases, we will be looking for panaceas — people must learn that as a rule they are not victims of something that comes from the *outside,* but, usually they are the offending culprits because of what they put or fail to put on the *inside* of their bodies.

I fully realize along with Dr. Alexander Bryce who said this: "Nothing offends patients more than to interfere with their habits of life, their desire is to break every known law of nature and when they get sick they accept complete absolution in a bottle or two of medicine — they merely want to be patched up sufficiently so they can go right back to their former habits of self indulgence in its various forms." Dr. Victor Heiser said: "Habit with him was all the test of truth — it must be right I've done it since my youth."

I'm sorry folks, that is not the way you either build or maintain or regain your health. Good health is an achievement — there are certain things you have to do about your daily habits of living and eating. Just in proportion as you do the good things, you will attain and maintain your physical future, your health, positive health, not merely the absence of disease. It is worth working for — Dr. Kirschner supplies you with a lifetime of valuable experiences — profit by them.

It has been my good fortune to see several of Dr. Kirschner's patients — I have talked to them, examined their mouths, teeth, bone and gums. I think I know what a healthy mouth looks like — I've been looking down in the mouth for over forty years and I saw health, radiant health where disease had been. The mouth is a barometer of health. I have many patients in my own practice who have followed good daily habits of living and I assure you there is no other way to positive health and a completely healthy body.

"Time is the essence — It's later than you think."

FRED D. MILLER, D.D.S., F.I.C.D.
Altoona, Penna.

Contents . . .

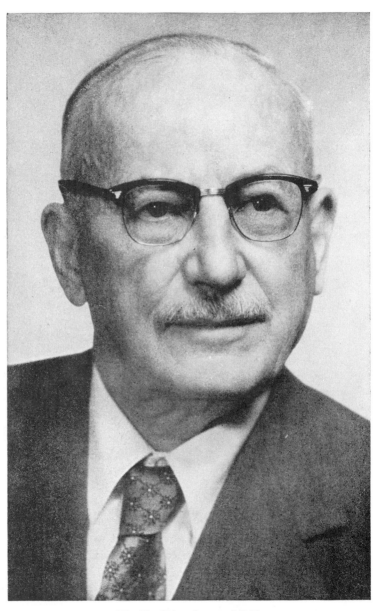

H. E. Kirschner, M.D.

Foreword . . .

THE TRUTHS contained in this book have been in the process of accumulation for the past fifty years, when the author studied the writings of a number of authorities on the subject of nutrition, and accepted this advice about maintaining good health — NO white flour, NO white sugar, NO tea or coffee, and NO alcohol or tobacco. How well this has paid off is shown by the present good health of the writer at the advanced age of eighty.

How many of you readers realize that *man* is the only animal that eats most of his food cooked? In prehistoric times, before man invented the "art" of cooking, the diet consisted largely of natural, raw, healthful foods — fruits, grains, nuts and vegetables. According to the Biblical record those early "pioneers" lived to be nearly a thousand years old! They picked their foods fresh from the orchard and garden, and ate them RAW. Can we today profit by their example?

During the past fifty years there have been many nutritionists who have been calling our attention to the value of RAW FOODS. But it is hard for man to give up lifelong practices and wrong habits of eating, even in the face of the multitudinous diseases so common today in the human race. According to one medical authority, "Never has culture been so advanced and complex as in our time, and never has there been so much mental disease, crime, insanity, and degeneracy!" Is natural food, unspoiled by processing and cooking the answer to our problem?

Some thirty years ago when friends of mine were traveling in Europe, the husband was taken very ill in Zurich, Switzerland. They inquired about a physician and were advised to go to the Bircher-Benner Sanatorium in that city.

7

The patient at first had some difficulty with the raw foods and juices which made up the treatment; but when all the poisons were eliminated from his body he made a very satisfactory recovery. On his return home he made me a present of a little booklet which described the method of taking the raw fruit, and the preparation of the vegetable juices. I became deeply interested in the therapeutic value of raw fruits and vegetable juices from my study of this little booklet.

Last year I went to Zurich, Switzerland, and enjoyed a stay at the Bircher-Benner Sanatorium, and observed the wonderful results from their methods of treatment of disease. Since this little book deals with the miraculous lifegiving force contained in fruit and vegetable juices, I want to quote from a book by Dr. Bircher-Benner — "The Essential Nature and Organization of Food Energy," published in 1936.

"Absorption and organization of sunlight, the essence of life, takes place almost exclusively within the plants. The organs of the plant are therefore, a kind of biological accumulation of light. They are the basis of what we call food, whence animal and human bodies derive their substance and energy. *Nutritional energy may thus be termed organized sunlight energy.* Hence sunlight is the driving force of the cells of our body."

This theory of "sunlight values" of food is supported by natural science and by experiments. I quote from the late Dr. Crile of Cleveland, Ohio, who told of "the striking example of physical property in living organisms, where radiation was demonstrated not only by photographs, but recorded by means of a photo-electric cell."

These observations have led our scientists to a new insight into the nature of FOOD ENERGY. Since both animal and man take food chiefly as a source of energy — this original food then conveys the energy of sunlight as organized by life.

In the past we have thought only in terms of *calories* in food. Now we have a far greater essential to consider. The raw fruit and vegetable juices contain this sunlight, and have been proven adequate for the RESTORATION of a diseased body to a condition of HEALTH.

This booklet will reveal to you what I have observed in recent years in the treatment of degenerative diseases through the use of fresh, raw juices. Much of the food eaten today has been so processed that little of value is left to keep our bodies in good condition. The raw juices are the LIFE BLOOD of the vegetables, and contain the vital enzymes and digestive factors so important to keep our bodies in a healthy condition.

In his book, "The New Food Therapy," Dietician Hans Anderson has this to say about raw vegetable juices. From page 23 I quote:

"Some practical experiments were described in the *American Journal of Physiology*, showing that raw vegetables require no digestion in the stomach compared with cooked foodstuffs, and that they remain in the stomach but a short time, similar to fruits. Raw vegetables, moreover, pass through the system largely as bulk, and are not fermentative, as are cooked foodstuffs, including vegetables. From such raw materials we receive LIVE FOOD minerals and vitamins unchanged by heating. LIVE VEGETABLE JUICES similar to those extracted from fresh fruits, require no work on the part of digestion, but are absorbed directly into the blood and are utilized by the weakest stomach."

Thanks to science and invention, today we have machines that make it a simple process to obtain the fresh, raw juices from our vegetables and fruits. These are in the form of *juicers* and *liquifiers*.

Nearly every day I am asked to explain the difference between a "juicer" and a "liquifier." When you liquify fruits or vegetables, you get the whole fruit or the whole vegetable, including the cellulose and the pulp. With the "juicer" the solids are eliminated, and you have the pure, concentrated juice *only,* containing the life-giving principles so essential in restoring our health.

Someone has aptly said: "You wouldn't think of eating a table full of raw vegetables — but your system may be starving for the minerals, vitamins and enzymes contained in a table full of raw vegetables!" By reducing that table full of life-giving vegetables to JUICE we have the answer to our problem. A good, reliable JUICER, therefore, is a gold mine investment in health.

The foregoing facts are emphasized by such well-known authorities on foods as R. D. Pope, M.D., and N. W. Walker, D.Sc., in their book "Raw Vegetable Juices," as follows: "To overcome the deficiency of live organic mineral salts in the human body, an abundant use of raw vegetable juices is essential because the digestive tract cannot assimilate the *volume of bulk* otherwise required by eating raw vegetables and fruits in sufficient quantities. As it is the chemistry of the individual that makes him what he is, both mentally and physically, the copious intake of raw vegetable juices will so re-chemicalize the body that NATURE will take care of the elimination of disease and the regeneration of the cells and the tissues."

This book has been written with only one purpose in mind — to share with you some of the remarkable experiences which through the years of my medical practice have transformed so many patients from sick, almost hopeless individuals, into happy, healthy men and women.

H. E. KIRSCHNER, M.D.

CHAPTER ONE

"THERE IS NO QUESTION THAT THE PEOPLE OF THIS NATION SHOULD BE EDUCATED TO CONSUME MORE OF THE NATURAL FOODS — AND TO STOP THE USE OF SO MANY UNWORTHY SUBSTITUTES. TODAY FOLKS ARE REALIZING THAT THE BEST MEDICINE IS FOOD!"

— Royal S. Copeland,
U. S. Senator, from New York.

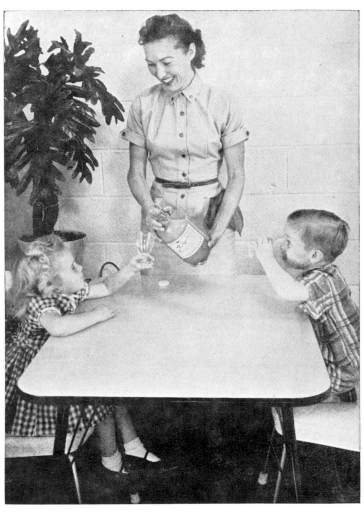

H. C. WHITE PHOTO

To guard against the hazards of malnutrition in her family, this young mother is shown giving her two children their daily ration of fresh, raw carrot juice. For the thrilling story of these youngsters, and their fight to conquer leukemia, see pages 49 and 50.

Health—A Personal Responsibility

HOW LONG before we learn that we have the same responsibility towards our bodies as the owner of a complex piece of machinery who must make sure it is correctly adjusted, lubricated, and in every way SAFEGUARDED? Often men are inclined to blatant boastfulness. "My health is GOOD! There is nothing wrong with ME!" *That person lives in a fool's paradise!* Often very successful men, very intelligent men in all other respects, ignore their HEALTH needs.

There was the case of an eminent lawyer who dropped dead at forty-eight. Famed far and wide for his knowledge of precedents and statutes, this so-called "wise man" paid absolutely no attention to his circulatory system and heart muscles, and the nutritional requirements of the same. Heart disease is the great killer. Approximately fifty percent of its victims die in the first attack. The survivors, learning through the devastating agony of that first attack, the penalty of indifference and ignorance, often recover and enjoy normal life for years — but only through a strict adherence to the sound principles of *correct nutrition.*

Research reveals that pyruvic acid in the blood stream is greatly increased when there is a deficiency of Vitamin B-1, which slows the action of the heart muscle to even one-half its normal rate. Present day nutritional knowledge emphasizes the importance of a daily consumption of liberal quantities of vegetables and fruits — two or three pounds a day being one of the best ways of obtaining adequate amounts of B-1.

13

Calcium, potassium, sodium and magnesium are vitally important to correct heart action. It is a well known fact that heart muscle may be kept alive for hours after removal from the body if supplied by circulation of blood or lymph adequately furnished with these vital elements. It is predicted that in a large measure, when nutritional knowledge is widespread ONLY THE IGNORANT WILL BE ILL. People will be as careful in selecting their food as they will in selecting materials for their homes. The house is built once, but human bodies are being constantly rebuilt.

Quoting a famous nutritionist: "It is now authoritatively established that by the simplest kind of diet correction, 90% of the tooth decay is preventable, and theoretically speaking 100% preventable. Also in the same manner, at least 50% of the so-called 'medical diseases' can be prevented or brought under control. The type of diets associated with dental degenerative diseases is similar to those associated with the so-called 'medical diseases' such as arthritis, arteriosclerosis, etc."

At the Governors' Conference, October 15-16, 1951, Dr. Michael J. Walsh, well-known Hollywood Nutritionist, made the following thought-provoking statement in his speech at the State Capitol in Sacramento. I quote:

"It is utterly hopeless, as well as catastrophic, to wait until disease happens and then furnish medical personnel to deal with it by treating symptoms — especially since there is growing evidence that degenerative disease is preventable before it happens. *The most important factor in the whole scheme of prevention is NUTRITION.*"

Dr. Robert McCarrison, speaking of a race of people in the remote Himalayas, living on what we would call a 'restricted diet', observed: "Magnificent physique — long life — unusually stable mentally — have no cancer — no heart disease — no rheumatism — no tuberculosis. A very frugal diet — vegetables — apricots — goat's milk — NO MEAT, except on feast days." These magnificent people are sometimes referred to as "The HEALTHY HUNZAS."

Vitamin "C" complex including P and K in some mysterious way is the "glue" which holds the cells of the tissues together. Total disintegration results when it is withdrawn — the blood vessels collapse. The process by which gristle becomes bone is halted, the nervous system becomes disorganized; there is a breakdown of the walls of the lungs; connective tissue disintegrates; little pools of stagnant blood are formed; bones soften because the process of calcification is halted; bacteria attack the organism. No resistance to tuberculosis results.

Approximately saturation is necessary to avoid such tragic consequences, — as pointed out by Dr. Rose in "Foundation of Nutrition," page 273, and Dr. Sherman's "Chemistry of Food and Nutrition."

Many people speak of food as "fuel" for the engine. As we have previously pointed out *food* does have a similar function in the body as fuel in the engine. It is a source of ENERGY. It is also the material from which the body is REBUILT — every portion of the body including the bony structures is in the process of wearing out, *Disintegration and rebuilding* are as NATURAL as day and night. Therefore foods must constantly furnish the elements of which the body is composed.

Why then, as intelligent people, do we not inform ourselves of these simple "facts of life" and supply ourselves with the component elements of the human body?

NOT TO KNOW YOUR BODY REQUIREMENTS AND SELECT YOUR FOOD TO MEET THESE REQUIREMENTS IS TO GAMBLE WITH YOUR MOST PRECIOUS POSSESSION — *HEALTH.*

Dr. McAlester tells us that "Science now offers to those who will use the newer knowledge of nutrition greater vigor and a high level of cultural attainment."

Let me repeat: Every part of the body from the toes to the hair on your head is constantly rebuilt. Loss of hair and teeth as well as a failure of the heart muscle points to one inescapable conclusion — faulty selection and utilization of food. Either carelessness or ignorance on this vital subject is SUICIDE!

Scientific knowledge is available to all — and the function of every food is so clearly understandable that to blunder on this point is inexcusable. What are the material things of life worth if you *lose your health?* What satisfaction is there in a beautiful home, or a Cadillac in the garage, if high blood pressure or hypertension make every day a PERIL? What wealth or material comfort can compensate for tortuous nights of arthritis pain, or the slow degeneration of tuberculosis?

BETTER SAFEGUARD YOUR HEALTH — IT IS YOUR GREATEST TREASURE IN THIS WORLD!

> "We squander Health
> In search of Wealth,
> We scheme and toil and save;
> Then squander Wealth
> In search of Health —
> And all we get's a grave.
> We live and boast of what we own,
> We die, and only get a stone."

CHAPTER TWO

"OF ALL THE MEDICINE CREATED
OUT OF THE EARTH, FOOD IS THE
CHIEF."

— *Sir Robert McCarrison, M.D.*

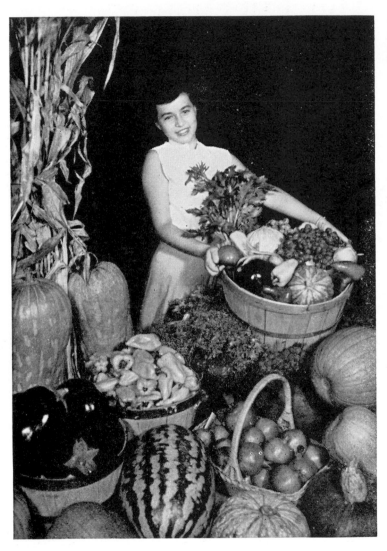

Mary Arena of Escondido, California proudly displays some of "Uncle Phil's" organically-grown produce at his popular "Roadside Market" on Highway 395.

The Function of Correct Nutrition

BEFORE WE go any further in our study, we should do some clear thinking, and come to an understanding of the function of CORRECT NUTRITION, and the function of MEDICINE.

Medicine in its practice is designed to meet an extremity — combat disease, destroy bacteria and virus, *kill* the killing disease. Then it must rely upon NATURE, using *all* the means at its disposal to REBUILD HEALTH.

In many cases, and, in the view of leading Bio chemists, who are the leaders and instructors of our doctors, most diseases are traced either directly or indirectly to POOR NUTRITION, or UNBALANCED NUTRITION.

The antiquated idea that the use of foods is only to provide energy, keep us warm, and enable us to work and play — overlooks the most important necessity of our bodies in these days of strenuous living.

As we have indicated in the preceding chapter, parts of the body are constantly aging — wearing out — and must be rebuilt. Not an entire part at a time being cast aside, as a worn-out bearing in a motor — although this actually happens with such items as hair and teeth. These are perhaps minor losses; but REAL TROUBLE comes when the heart muscle or an important gland wears out!

Proper nutrition supplies energy not only to the brain and muscles, but must also provide the "building blocks" to restore the worn-out cells of every part of the body — thus constantly renewing its very structure.

Authorities tell us that while food provides these "building blocks" in the form of protein or energy from sugars or starches; in order to utilize these elements we must have an abundance of vitamins, minerals and enzymes. Certain vitamins are known today, but many are yet unknown — but ALL ARE NECESSARY. All these precious minerals and vitamins are found in a balanced utilizable form in vegetables. All doctors agree that we need raw green and yellow vegetables in far greater quantities than any of us consume.

Dr. Henry Sherman, who is widely quoted by medical men and nutritionists, and who is perhaps the world's greatest authority on the vital subject of foods, states:

"When nutritional knowledge is sufficiently widespread, people will consume up to three pounds of green and yellow vegetables and fruits daily." And then he adds: "The MORE the BETTER!"

Why should we get our vitamins and minerals from raw vegetables and fruits in preference to any other way? You need much raw food daily in the diet. WHY? Because the enzymes are produced by the glands from food elements, and good health is impossible when the enzyme producing glands atrophy. Heed this important fact. The elements from which enzymes are produced are destroyed at 126 degrees Fahrenheit. You need much live, raw food daily in order to supply the glands with a reserve of these essential, vital elements.

WHY USE JUICES? Why not just eat the raw vegetables? As we have indicated in the previous chapter, for optimal health you need far more than you could possibly eat. The stomach just couldn't handle that much bulk. Then too, if modern research is correct, the power to break down the cellular structure of raw vegetables, and assimilate the precious elements they contain, even in the healthiest individual is only fractional — not more than 35%, and in the less healthy, down to 1%.

In the form of juice, these same individuals assimilate up to 92% of these elements. The juice of the plant, like the blood of the body contains all the elements that build and nourish. It is a well-known fact that all foods must become liquid before they can be assimilated.

It is also an established fact that many of the elements of the plant can be obtained by eating the animal that lives on the plant; that is if we eat the glandular part of the animal in which these precious food elements are stored. But as you can readily see, that method is getting our minerals and vitamins and enzymes "second-hand"! Why not *eat the plant* that builds the body structure of the animal? Raw fruit and vegetable juices enable us to do just that, and we get our vital elements in their entirety — unchanged and unspoiled by cooking.

FOOD FOR THOUGHT

The important role of minerals in our effort to maintain optimal health is emphasized in a recent report made by Dr. Tom Douglas Spies at the Annual Meeting of the American Medical Association as follows:

"All diseases are *caused* by chemicals, and all diseases can be *cured* by chemicals. All the chemicals used by the body (except for the oxygen which we breathe and the water which we drink) are taken in through food. *If we only knew enough, all diseases could be prevented, and could be cured, through proper nutrition.* . . .

"As tissues become damaged, they lack the chemicals of good nutrition, they tend to become old. They lack what I call 'tissue integrity.' There are people of 40 whose brains and arteries are senile. If we can help the tissues repair themselves by correcting nutritional deficiencies, we can make old age wait."

———————◇———————

Dr. Risser, noted Pasadena Bone Specialist states: "INFANTILE PARALYSIS can be prevented by a diet rich in vitamin C."

Dr. Norman Joliffe, in making experiments with five healthy volunteers, found that after only four days without Vitamin B-1 electro-cardiograms showed the hearts were abnormal.

———————◇———————

British Report on Juice Therapy

The British Government, having assumed the responsibility for the people's health, is relying upon every means that is successful to obtaining that end. Therefore, they have made ample tests on the value of vegetable juices.

Herein are the facts ascertained by the "Ministry of Health and Public Health Service Laboratory" of Great Britain, which set forth that to obtain best results, juices should be used immediately as storage losses were great.

"The sources of the essential amino acids, the cell building factors, are destroyed by heat and processing and not obtainable in foods thus prepared; juices, therefore, are the only means practical to get these *rebuilding factors.*

"Juices are valuable in relief of hypertension, cardiovascular and kidney diseases and obesity. Good results have also been obtained in rheumatic, degenerative and toxic states. Juices have all-around protective action. Good results can be obtained in large amounts up to one litre daily in treatment of peptic ulceration, also in treatment of chronic diarrhea, colitis and toxemia of gastro and intestinal origin.

"The high buffering capacities of the juices reveal that they are very valuable in the treatment of hyperchlorhydria. Milk has often been used for this purpose, but spinach juices, juices of cabbage, kale and parsley were far superior to milk for this purpose." (Acting as a sort of gyroscope in balancing the alkali and the acid condition of the system.)

CHAPTER THREE

"LEAVE YOUR DRUGS IN THE
CHEMIST'S POT IF YOU CAN HEAL
THE PATIENT WITH FOOD!"
— *Hippocrates, the Father of Medicine.*

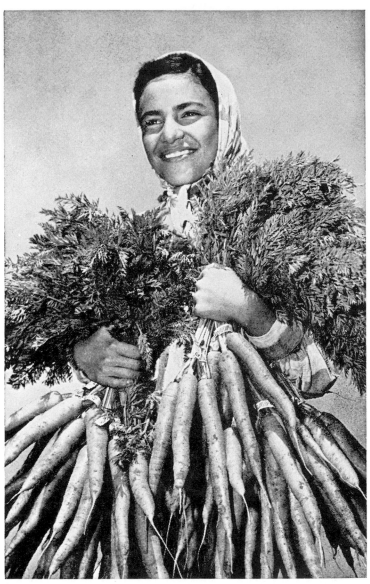

California carrots by the armload — soon to be transformed into "liquid gold" — are helping to "re-build" sick bodies and bring them back to more abundant health and renewed joy of living.

A "Golden" Nutritional Discovery

WHEN the writer went off to Medical College sixty-one years ago, he was a sickly young man of eighteen years. He had worked hard earning money to go to college. He had suffered much from stomach trouble, which later on developed into a duodenal ulcer and necessitated an operation at the Mayo Clinic.

Having this ill health at college, the writer read every book he could find on health and diet, and finally found the plan outlined in the Foreword, plus a diet containing plenty of fruits and vegetables and *little* meat.

The author now finds that he enjoys better health, and is in better physical condition than any of the few survivors from his medical class of fifty-seven years ago.

The great value of fresh vegetable juices was again brought to my attention by a Mrs. Hogle, of Salt Lake City. This woman had been ill for a long time, and had consulted many physicians for an ailment of her stomach accompanied with feeble digestion and other intestinal complaints.

The advice given her was to eat nourishing food, after many efforts with drugs had failed. One day there was a rap on Mrs. Hogle's door and an elderly man asked her if he could interest her in some fresh carrot juice, telling her how his health had been restored through its use.

Mrs. Hogle was desperate enough to try anything, so she arranged for this man to deliver his fresh carrot juice to her each day. It was not long before her digestion and elimination improved, and she became interested in helping others by devising a machine to cut up the carrots by electricity, and a press with which to extract the juice.

Later on, Mrs. Hogle came to California to visit relatives, and when I showed an interest in using the juice to treat tuberculosis patients, she presented me with one of her machines. I had a gardener who grew carrots for the market, and every day my helpers made large quantities of carrot juice, which I used very successfully in treating not only tuberculosis, but other chronic ailments.

Then came the climax to my interest in this new way of treating illnesses that failed to respond to the use of drugs. I was placed in charge of some 200 tuberculosis patients for the County of Los Angeles. (Olive View Sanitorium — Outside Service.) The daily diet of these patients consisted largely of macaroni and spaghetti and other starches and over-cooked food.

Some of these patients had spent nine long years on their backs with very little progress toward recovery. I had a small ranch where I grew alfalfa, parsley and spinach. Every day the leaves of these greens were juiced, and a glass of this "green drink" daily soon changed the progress of these patients to that of recovery. In fact patients who had been considered hopeless were able to be out of bed in six to eight months. With my private patients, where this mixture could be combined with fresh carrot juice the improvement was even more rapid.

Another outstanding "case history" that deepened my interest in the life-giving qualities of fresh, raw carrot juice, was that of Mr. B. of Oregon. Having some business in Northern California, I decided to get from Mr. B firsthand the details of his dramatic experience with the use of carrot juice, for I had heard much about this man during the preceding year.

Upon reaching Mr. B's home, I found him to be a man of sixty-four years. Although he was born in Texas, he had lived for twenty-three years in Baltimore before coming West to Oregon ten years ago. His family was short-lived. Mr. B's father died at the age of forty, and his mother at sixty-four. He had three brothers, all of whom are dead; also a sister who died of cancer at the age of forty-five.

Mr. B's illness started in 1948. However, for some fifteen years prior to that time, he suffered with terrible pains in his abdomen in the region of his stomach. He was treated by many physicians for stomach trouble, but medicine did not seem to reach his ailment. . . . In 1948 he passed blood in his urine and suffered from a breaking out of warts on his head.

Inasmuch as he was a newcomer in the city where he was living, Mr. B asked several people to give him the name of a good physician upon whom he might call. They all recommended the same one. . . . The physician whom he contacted made no examination, merely questioned him — then burned his warts with nitric acid, and for the bleeding told him to take three or four drops of turpentine on a spoonful of sugar three times a day. The bleeding stopped for the time being. But in two months the bleeding started again, and the same treatment was prescribed.

After seven months, Mr. B went to another physician, who, upon hearing his story, sent him to a specialist in a neighboring city. Following an examination, the specialist advised an operation on the next day, to which Mr. B agreed. A growth, which proved to be cancerous, was removed from Mr. B's bladder.

Four months later, another operation was performed on this man, and some radium seeds were implanted in his bladder where the growth had been removed. Then three months after the implanting of the radium seeds, he went to a veteran's hospital. The physician who now treated him told Mr. B's wife that if he lived the year out, he would be fortunate.

I saw a photograph of Mr. B's left kidney which was removed in 1949. The picture showed that the kidney was enlarged to twice its normal size, and at least a dozen areas of cancer could be seen on its surface.

Up to the time he started drinking vegetable juice in 1951, Mr. B had gone through some forty operations and examinations of his bladder. In health, this man weighed 183 pounds, but a short time after going to the hospital and being operated on, his weight was down to 128 pounds — a loss of 55 pounds.

At first Mr. B drank only a glassful of carrot juice a day, and he didn't see any beneficial results. But in 1953, when he increased the amount to two quarts a day, he noticed marked improvement in his strength and health. Soon he was able to start work selling juicers. His weight increased to 155 pounds — a gain of 27 pounds.

Now at the age of 64, Mr. B never has a cold, and for one who was so ill for such a length of time, he enjoys remarkable vitality, full capacity for work, and enjoyment of life.

WHAT AMERICA NEEDS

Senator Thomas C. Desmond, of New York, Member of the Joint Legislative Committee on Nutrition, declares: "America desperately needs leadership in the field of NUTRITION. — Teach us what we need to know about our Diets. 'Strengthen our FOOD that it may give its strength to ourselves and our children,' is the prayer of the American people."

CHAPTER FOUR

"NO PHARMACIST WILL EVER COMPOUND A PILL, PATENT MEDICINE OR DRUG THAT CAN COMPARE IN CURATIVE VALUE WITH THE VALUE FOUND IN UNCOOKED, PURE FRUIT AND VEGETABLE JUICES."

— *The Joy of Living.*

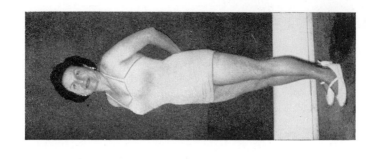

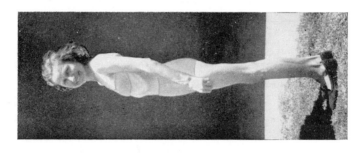

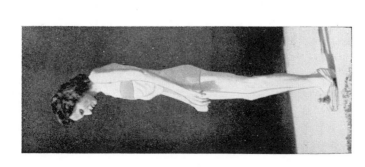

REMARKABLE IMPROVEMENT . . . Photograph at left shows patient at beginning of carrot juice regimen when her weight was less than 65 pounds. Center picture was taken five months later, weight had increased to 94 pounds. Photograph at right shows patient as she is today with normal weight of 135 pounds.

Therapeutic Use of Carrot Juice

FROM my reading of old health books I find that the use of carrots and carrot juice as a therapeutic agent is an ancient practice. A book published in Germany in 1840 speaks highly of the healing properties of this golden vegetable in treating disease.

The strong antiseptic qualities of carrots was referred to in various English publications. And many years ago the great Professor Metchnikoff made the discovery that the stool of rabbits fed on carrots lost its odor and had become free from putrefactive germs.

There are health resorts in Europe where patients are fed carrots three times a day in some form, as part of their treatment. Miracles of restoration follow in the wake of this simple therapeutic agency.

Recently the following remarkable "case history" came to my attention, which confirmed the work that I did twenty years ago in treating tuberculosis patients with alfalfa, parsley, carrot, and other juices.

When calling on a friend near my home I was asked to visit a place where carrot juice was being made; a large amount of which was delivered by a local dairy to its customers.

The friend wanted to know if the juice was being produced under sanitary conditions, and if I could recommend its use after learning where the carrots were grown and the care that was taken in cleaning them and processing the juice.

My visit was a great success. While visiting the plant I learned why Mr. and Mrs. X were engaged in their present work. Their breathtaking story is little short of miraculous.

Mrs. X was born in California in 1911. She had spent most of her life on a farm; but had never cared for milk. Her family, like so many other rural American families, lived on starches (refined), fried potatoes and fatty meat. Fruit was a luxury. She was married at the age of sixteen. and from then on had better food.

After an automobile accident, approximately eighteen years ago, Mrs. X's nearly fatal illness started. Within a few days she became subject to nervousness accompanied with a severe attack of jaundice.

I saw by records of her illness in 1941 at a well-known clinic, where a diagnosis of gall bladder disease was made, and that she had lost sixteen pounds. She did not improve with extensive medication, and became so ill that she was placed in a Sanatorium where she had intravenous medication for three weeks.

In spite of all that could be done, Mrs. X continued to lose weight, and at one time vomited for twelve days with an additional loss of twelve pounds. Her weight, normally 135 pounds, was now below 65 pounds. The diagnosis of splenic leukemia had been made by three different physicians.

Becoming desperate, Mrs. X consulted a woman who had studied medicine in Europe, and who had a thorough training in the use of raw fruit and vegetable juices in the treatment of disease. This woman claimed she had been cured of cancer by carrot and other juices after medicine had failed.

Before starting on the carrot juice diet the patient (Mrs. X) had no control of her bowels for one year. Her condition was so desperate that she could only take the carrot juice by the spoonful. Gradually it was increased to an eight-ounce glass every twenty-four hours. Finally she was taking one gallon of juice per day!

No other liquid food or medication passed Mrs. X's lips for eighteen months! During the first two months she had a stormy time with reactions — hemorrhages from the bowels, and other alarming symptoms — and NO GAIN in weight. Then all at once the course of her disease miraculously changed, and she gained one pound a week steadily until her normal weight of 135 pounds was reached. (See accompanying photographs.)

Another symptom that had bothered her a great deal before starting the carrot juice therapy was arthritic pains in her joints. She could not even use her hands. This condition rapidly disappeared with the improvement in her general health.

Her first solid food after eighteen months on carrot juice was liquified peaches (ripe from the tree), Romaine lettuce (only the juice), celery, pears, dates, and honey. Now her diet consists of carrot juice all day, and after work in the evening a large salad of raw vegetables with avocado, sunflower or sesame seeds, or a few nuts.

For the past nine and a half years the patient has been working hard from twelve to sixteen hours per day, and on her feet constantly. Her health is perfect, and she has been free from colds.

When one can eliminate a serious condition that took over ten years to develop, simply by drinking carrot juice over a period of eighteen months, this health method certainly deserves the attention of the medical profession.

Hans Anderson, noted dietician, tells the story of a woman who at the age of seventy-two was suffering from cancer of the abdomen. Because of her advanced age she had been looking forward to an early grave. "We were requested to advise her what to eat. We informed her that in cases of advanced tissue degeneration the only biological approach would be for a rejuvenation and reconstruction of the entire being. For this purpose, *live food juices* had proved to be a wise means for the infusion of *new life* and strength into both blood and tissue.

"The case under consideration accepted our plan for rejuvenation through a system of feeding on *live food juices* and whole foodstuffs. The woman made a splendid recovery, and is still active at the age of ninety-four!"

———————◇———————

MORE FOOD FOR THOUGHT

Dr. Rhinehart, University of California, states "NEARLY EVERYONE TAKES HIS HEALTH FOR GRANTED.". . . Those who become hopelessly ill exclaimed a short while before: 'I am healthy — my heart is strong.' On becoming ill they wail: 'I would give anything in the world to get my health back!' "

———————◇———————

Burdensome, excessive fat, so harmful to heart and kidneys, is the result of Vitamin Deficiency. Starches and sugars are not transformed into energy. A long waistline, scientists inform us, means a shortened life-line. AVOID OVERWEIGHT!

———————◇———————

"It is a safe rule to increase your fruits and vegetables and juices and cut down on your starches and sweets, milk, and meats, for good health and longevity," says Dr. Lloyd C. Shanklin.

———————◇———————

"Since we are part of Nature, and subject to her rules and laws, we ought to be observant of her methods in our search for Truth and the answers to our problems."

CHAPTER FIVE

"FOR IMPARTING VITALITY AND BUILDING UP RESISTANCE TO DISEASE, RAW JUICES HAVE NO EQUAL, AND SHOULD FORM PART OF THE DAILY DIETARY OF YOUNG AND OLD ALIKE."

— *Lawrence Armstrong,*
Famous Australian Food-Scientist.

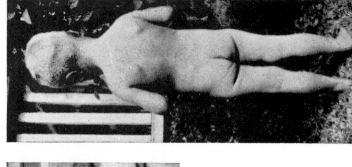

No. 3 ... Miraculous change in youngster's physical condition in less than two years

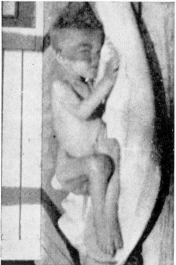

No. 1 ... Child at two and one-half years, unable to stand alone and weighing only 16½ pounds.

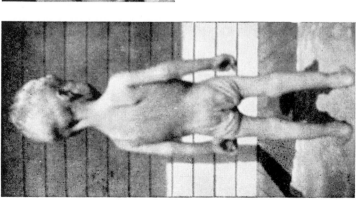

No. 2 ... After approximately 10 months on raw juices child is able to stand alone and

The Story of a
Modern Miracle

THE REACTIONS to my story about the woman who lived eighteen months on no food other than raw carrot juice have been most interesting. Whenever I tell the story I am greeted with such remarks as: "This is impossible! Surely she had other food.". . . "What about the amino acids?" . . . Where did her protein come from?" . etc., etc.

If my friends are surprised and skeptical about the story of Mrs. X, the "carrot juice woman," I wonder what they will say when I tell the story of the man who lived for four and one-half years on nothing but carrot juice and the solids from goat whey, and cured himself of cancer; or about the woman who cured her arthritis with carrot and other juices, and who today lives entirely on juices — and works hard!

But recently, an even greater miracle of restoration through Juice Therapy has been brought to my attention. A letter, accompanied with photographs (see illustrations), was received from Mr. and Mrs. N, of Kansas. In photo No. 1 you see a baby two and one-half years old, who weighed only 16½ pounds. This child was allergic to milk and all animal products. The distraught parents could find no food or medicine that the child could take. He was so weak he couldn't even turn over in bed, and the end was only a question of days.

Fortunately for all concerned the mother had the good sense to start the sick child on raw, fresh juices — carrot juice predominating, with the result that at last the child started to improve. In the second photo, the child could stand alone, but notice the folds in the skin of his buttocks. In the third photograph you will note what a wonderful change has taken place in the child's physical condition. In less than two years on the juice diet, the little fellow was perfectly well, and normal in every way.

All this happened eighteen years ago, but the letter from the child's parents makes it sound as if it had occurred only yesterday. Here is the parents' remarkable story:

"Our boy at first was what everyone called a healthy child. At fourteen months he suddenly became very sick, and soon went into convulsions. These lasted almost continuously for eight hours before getting them stopped. After the doctor ordered him to the hospital he was given a large hypo deep into the thigh. There were no more convulsions, but he was entirely unconscious for several days. In about a week the doctor pronounced him well, and told us to feed him plenty of good nourishing food, which we did. But every few weeks he had a 'sick spell' and was seriously threatened with more convulsions. He was very nervous and did a lot of jerking in his sleep for over a year. He was taken to perhaps a dozen different doctors, and each diagnosed his trouble differently. One doctor put him on an entire milk diet, but he grew worse and lost weight.

"When he was a little over two years old we thought our child was improving, but to our surprise his plumpness was a bad case of edema. He was sick and cried continuously. He couldn't eat, he couldn't digest or assimilate his food. For over two and one-half years he never had a normal bowel movement. He passed large quantities of mucous, and had large hemorrhoids.

"At this time (two and one-half years old) he was in bed and remained there for five months. He became so sick and helpless he could not turn over in bed. He was on the road to the grave, and our friends offered their sympathy. He became skin and bones and weighed 16½ pounds. The doctor's general opinion was that he had tuberculosis of the colon, and probably would never get well. He also said if he should improve, he likely would have epilepsy the rest of his life.

"We live in Kansas about 300 miles east of Denver. We heard of a doctor in that city who used natural methods of healing. Through correspondence the doctor helped us to realize that we were overfeeding our boy. His diet was cut down to a few ounces daily of fruit and vegetable juices, and a very small amount of broth and toast.

"After about eight or ten months our son had gained about two pounds, but could not walk across the floor. . . . We built a house trailer, and by following God's leading started for California to seek further help. In California we met a doctor who gave us a basic diet of raw fruit and vegetable juices — raw carrot juice was used more than any other juice. We also used some fresh juice from Thompson's grapes. Honey was used as an energy food.

"After six or eight months on nothing but raw juices, our boy made remarkable improvement. His bowels began to move naturally after each meal. His hemorrhoids and mucous disappeared. He now began to demand some solid foods such as salads and cooked vegetables. No cereals or meats were used.

"At four years and two months our child weighed thirty-nine pounds; played all the time with other children, and slept like a log at night.

"At the time of this writing our son is twenty-two years old. He is enjoying perfect health. He never had any tooth caries until he left home and lived in a college dormitory where he could not get proper foods. He is six feet tall, and has never been sick a day in his life after his recovery in his early years. We consider his miraculous recovery largely due to the use of 'live foods' in the form of juice — CARROT being the *foundation* of all."

In the following pages of this booklet, I have other stories of the wonderful healing properties of fresh, raw vegetable juices, but none are more miraculous than the story of this young man from Kansas.

LONG LIFE

Long life can be enjoyed — not endured. The research of Dr. Sherman of Columbia University proves that life can be considerably prolonged, but what is more important, the prime of life may be extended and made vigorous by correct nutrition.

On this point of lengthening the life span, Dr. Jonathan Forman, Editor of the *Ohio State Medical Journal,* has this to say: "It is possible for human beings to maintain perfect health from the cradle to the grave. . . . This should be the goal of each one of us. In doing so we would likewise greatly lengthen our life span. Not only would we add years to our lives but, what is more important, we would add life to our years. . . .

"The most important factor in the maintenance of optimal health is the highest state of nutrition. The maintenance of the best possible state of nutrition depends upon GOOD FOOD. The quality of one's food depends upon the selection of excellent foodstuffs, which have not been spoiled in the harvest, storage, processing, preserving, preparing, or serving. . . .

"Once Americans begin eating foods grown on soil containing ALL the essential mineral elements, unspoiled in its processing and preparation, disease will practically vanish, the normal life span will be about 120 years, our national disposition will improve. We will have no cause to fear old age."

CHAPTER SIX

"THE FOOD QUESTION IS IN-
FINITELY THE MOST IMPORTANT
PROBLEM OF THE PRESENT DAY. —
AND IF PROPERLY DEALT WITH
MUST RESULT IN THE DISAPPEAR-
ANCE OF THE VAST BULK OF DIS-
EASE, MISERY, AND DEATH."

— *Sir Arbuthnot Lane, M.D.*

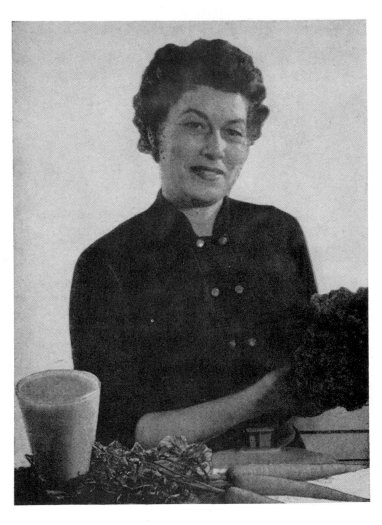

H. C. WHITE PHOTO

The narrator of the following remarkable "case history" is here shown in action, demonstrating the preparation of live food juices. In addition to caring for her family, this busy housewife spends much time helping other sufferers, who like herself, are afflicted with serious physical disorders. In spite of her handicap, she even gives demonstration-lectures on the benefits of juice therapy to large audiences. (From an unretouched photograph.)

An Amazing
Case History

(As Told by the Patient)

IN FEBRUARY, 1956, at the urgent request of my parents I went to my doctor for a complete medical checkup. At the time I didn't feel ill, and was holding down a full-time job in addition to caring for my family. However, there were symptoms that indicated that all was not well. I was emaciated, and suffered from discoloration of the skin in the upper portion of my body. I was also subject to violent vomiting spells, headache, and backache. All these I attributed to overwork. At this time I was forty-one years old, and the mother of four living sons.

The results of the tests and X-rays showed me in apparent good health, with the exception of my right kidney. But as the kidney was still functioning, the doctor advised against immediate surgery. He felt that I might "get by" for at least another year before having it removed. He reported that I had probably had the condition for two or three years, and assured me that he would not let things get out of control.

In November, 1956, I returned to the Clinic for another checkup. The results of the dye test and the X-rays showed that both kidneys were now affected. I was sent to one of the best Urologists in Los Angeles County, who put me in the hospital within a matter of hours. Cystoscope. X-ray and other tests indicated immediate surgery — if possible.

After hours of physical and mental torture, I was told that surgery was absolutely *impossible,* as both kidneys were now barely functioning, and much of each kidney was already destroyed. The X-rays showed that the kidneys were collapsing and in a state of rapid disintegration. The doctors informed me that I had a rare and fatal kidney disease called "Pyo-nephrosis," for which there was no known cure. When I inquired how long they figured I had to live, I was told that with God's help, plenty of rest, a rigid diet, and if I could respond favorably to all known antibiotics, perhaps I might live a year.

On November 26th, I was put on a rigid diet, including one small glass of milk, some sweets, green leafy vegetables, yellow vegetables, tomatoes, celery and rice. But, unfortunately this diet did not seem to help. My weight dropped to 98 pounds. I suffered agony from bloating and edema, and often was confined to my bed with severe hemorrhaging. By December I was suffering so much pain, it was almost unbearable, and we sought the advice of many Urologists and surgeons, including those from the Mayo Clinic. All these specialists confirmed the original diagnosis. None gave any hope of recovery.

I now began failing so fast I could scarcely believe it was really *me*. My strength was ebbing daily, and the hemmorrhages became more frequent and severe. I began to pass pieces of kidney tissue, and pain racked my body day and night. Each urine specimen, taken three times a week, showed a more alarming condition than the one previous. Pus and blood were present in ever increasing amounts. I could stay only three days at a time on any one antibiotic, and then was switched to another. Yet my life was slowly but surely ebbing away.

By the last week in April my condition became extremely critical. I could scarcely say more than a few words and would be completely out of breath, due to a lock of oxygen in my system. Breathing became so difficult that I found myself fighting for every breath. The doctors told my family I'd be lucky if I lived three weeks.

Then one day I met a very dear friend whom I had not seen in eighteen years. At first she did not recognize me, and was shocked beyond words at my physical condition. One of her first questions was: "Lola, have you ever tried raw juice therapy?" I didn't even know what she was talking about. Then she proceeded to relate many interesting stories about the therapeutic value of live food juices. She asked me if I had ever read a book on this subject by a physician in nearby Monrovia. I said, "No." She immediately left the house and rushed to the nearest Health Food Store, and was soon back with a copy of the book. She begged me to read the miraculous experience of Mrs. X; of the little boy from Nebraska, and other thrilling case histories found in "Live Food Juices."

I read the book, and was deeply impressed with its "common sense" approach to the problem of disease — its *cause* and *cure*. I felt, however, that I personally was beyond the point of being helped. But my mother and father and family insisted that I give this raw juice therapy a "try." After all, I had nothing to lose and everything to gain in following the instructions found in this new book.

I started immediately, drinking one gallon of fresh, raw carrot juice daily, and a half gallon of the author's therapeutic "green drink," made from green leafy vegetables, including alfalfa, parsley, dandelion, water-cress, mint, beet greens, etc. (See formula on page 118.)

When I began drinking these fresh, raw juices, I refused all other medication — all hypos, all antibiotics, and all food in bulk form, either cooked or raw. Nothing passed my lips but fresh, raw juices, extracted daily by my husband. Many of my friends thought that by discarding all medicine and cooked foods, I'd surely die.

To make a long story short, three days after taking *absolutely nothing* but the raw juices, I began to breathe easier and deeper. I was greatly encouraged and could notice improvement daily. I could talk for five or ten minutes without losing my breath; my heart improved, and the "gushing" noise in my ears stopped. I could also move my legs in bed without help.

On the sixth day, I asked my husband to help me out of bed; for I felt I could now stand on my feet. I had to insist, and he finally consented to let me try to stand alone — and I did! On the eighth day I took my first steps alone in many weeks. Then on the tenth day, as is usual in cases of extreme toxemia, I suffered a terrific "reaction." With almost unbearable pain in my back, accompanied by alarming hemorrhaging, I was about to be taken back to the hospital, when suddenly the bleeding stopped, and plans to rush me to the hospital were cancelled.

While I was very weak following that terrible hemorrhage, I was not unduly alarmed. I had been told that many who are in a most critical condition, experience some pretty "rough" reactions during the early stages of the raw juice therapy. Within three hours after the violent hemorrhage (which, by the way, was my last) all pain in by back and body began to subside, and the following day miraculously vanished. I could scarcely believe it myself! To be able to rest — no fever — no pain — it was like a dream!

This is April, 1958, and my condition is steadily improving. My weight is now back to normal; I continue daily on my gallon of carrot juice and one quart of the "green drink." Since the last of October, I've eaten a small vegetable salad, and some fresh fruits daily. It has now been more than a year since any meat or animal products or cooked foods have passed my lips. I am able to do a great deal of my own house-work now. Of course, I must go *slow* and not become unduly fatigued.

O, it is so wonderful and so gratifying to be on my feet again after being so near to death's door! I am so grateful for the knowledge I have obtained — that proper *diet* is the greatest single health factor. There can be no substitute for live foods, naturally grown, to nourish and purify a polluted blood stream, or to regenerate and rebuild the tissues of a sick, broken body. I KNOW, because this miracle, thank God, has happened to ME!

CHAPTER SEVEN

"I BELIEVE I WOULD NOT BE FAR
OUT OF THE WAY TO SAY THAT
DIET MAY BE SAID TO BE A FACTOR
IN EVERY DISEASE TO WHICH MAN
IS HEIR."

— *Harvey W. Wiley, M.D.*

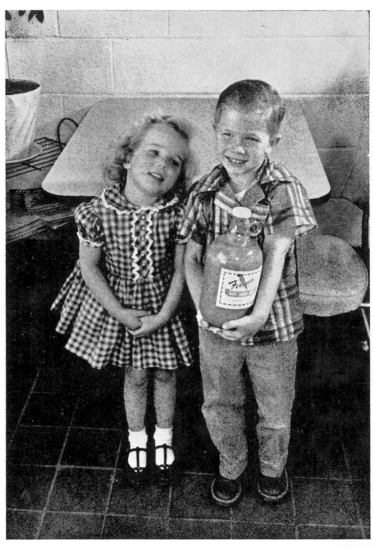

"Love that carrot juice!" Here on the right, holding the big jug of Ferraro's carrot juice, which he has taken from birth, is the little fellow who was born with leukemia. At the age of five there are no traces of this dread disease. His little four-year-old sister is also a confirmed "drinker" of live food juices.

Leukemia Arrested With Raw Juices

THE STORY I am about to relate is one of the most remarkable that has been brought to my attention during more than fifty years of medical practice. It involves the "case histories" of three children — all from one family — one of which developed leukemia soon after birth; the second child, which was born with leukemia, and the third, which was given carrot juice immediately after birth, and has remained in a condition of perfect health.

The first child, a baby girl, was born in 1951 At the time of birth the doctor referred to her as his "prize baby." Apparently she was perfectly normal at that time. This beautiful little girl was dark-complexioned like her father, but her color soon began to fade, and after two months she was so pale the parents became alarmed and consulted their physician. The doctor ordered an immediate blood count, which revealed the sad fact that this baby girl was suffering from leukemia. She was taken to the hospital, and there within the space of five and one-half days she was given twenty-five blood transfusions. But all these super-human efforts to save the child were fruitless, and the little girl died at the age of three months.

The second child, a boy, was born in 1953. An examination of the child's blood revealed the terrifying fact that this second baby was *born with leukemia!* The baby's doctor had become acquainted with the remarkable experience of Mrs. Catherine Ferraro, who had recovered from splenic leukemia by taking large quantities of fresh, raw carrot juice daily. He was determined to save this second baby, if possible, by the same means. He immediately contacted Mrs. Ferraro by telephone, and arranged for her to bring two quarts of carrot juice to the hospital each day. Although the Ferraros were not in the carrot juice business at the time, they graciously responded to this emergency, and when the baby went home the carrot juice therapy was continued.

It is interesting to note that during the first three months of this baby's life, NO OTHER FOOD was allowed. After three months, however, other foods were added to his diet, including both fruits and vegetables. Did this simple raw juice therapy work? Much to the joy and satisfaction of every one concerned, at the end of one year the blood count was normal. There was no evidence of leukemia! The carrot juice had evidently performed a miracle in restoring the child's diseased bloodstream to a normal healthy condition.

Today, at the age of five, with the exception of some occasional bronchial asthma, the little fellow is apparently in perfect health. He continues to take his daily ration of carrot juice. He also drinks lots of citrus juices, of which he is very fond. His weight is 48 pounds.

The third child, a beautiful little girl, was born in 1954. Blood tests made at the time of birth showed no evidence of leukemia. The blood count was normal. This favorable condition was no doubt largely due to the fact that the mother drank quantities of carrot juice regularly throughout her pregnancy. Having become enthusiastic "converts" to the raw juice therapy, the parents weren't taking any chances, and the third child was also given nothing but carrot juice for the first three months after birth. Now, at the age of four she still takes two glasses of carrot juice per day, and the two youngsters consume a gallon of juice a week. (See illustration.) They are now the "picture" of vibrant good health.

What more convincing evidence could anyone find, showing the powerful remedial effects of the raw juice therapy than that which we have noted above? I doubt if there has ever been a comparable case recorded in the annals of medical history.

Arthritis Responds to Live Juice Therapy

SEVERAL MONTHS ago my attention was called to the remarkable case history of Mrs. A. Her experience is so typical of the healing virtues of live food juices in the incidence of arthritis — one of the great curses of our modern civilization — that I wish to share her experience with my readers. Here is her story as she told it to me:

"For more than twenty years I was afflicted with arthritis. At the age of nineteen the first distressing symptoms appeared. It started in my right foot, and in a matter of days the joints of my knees, elbows, wrists and fingers were affected. I was in constant pain. I went to the doctors for help; but they told me there was no known cure for arthritis. They tried to relieve the pain, but their efforts helped very little. There were days when I didn't suffer so much, but the pain never left my body.

"At the age of twenty-six I developed inflammatory arthritis. I was now completely helpless and unable to move. The pain was unbearable, and I hurt so I didn't see how I could live. To help relieve the excruciating pain, the doctors gave me morphine. As time passed, other things happened to my body. My heart beat so fast at times it seemed to take my breath away.

"Then five years ago (1954), I heard about the therapeutic value of raw fruit and vegetable juices. I had tried so many things over the years, all of which had failed to bring relief, I was a bit skeptical that such simple measures could do anything to help *me*. I saw no harm, however, in grasping at this "last straw" as it were, and I decided to give the juices a "try."

"When I began to take the fruit and vegetable juices, I gave up all cooked food. I ate no meat. I drank no water. I also gave up sugar, salt, and all condiments. I drank two quarts of carrot juice a day, and one pint of fresh grapefruit juice, and one pint of fresh celery juice. I also took small amounts of beet and parsley juice.

"The radical change in my dietary habits brought on the usual severe "reactions," and as the cleansing process progressed, I suffered from gas and running off of the bowels, and other unpleasant symptoms. In spite of all this, however, I continued with the juice diet, and soon I began to feel better.

"At the end of eight months, all pain had left my body, and the crippling deformities that usually accompany arthritis, disappeared. For the first time, in more than twenty years I was free from suffering. I discovered the wonderful fact that I was now a *well woman!* I had worn glasses most of my life; but after one year on the juice diet, I tossed out my "bi-focals." My eyesight had somehow been miraculously restored to normal, and glasses were now, for me, a thing of the past.

"Today, my diet consists of only raw fruits and vegetables, plus the fruit and vegetable juices. I still drink at least two quarts of carrot juice a day, and a pint of citrus juice, plus one avocado and some kelp. After all those years of inactivity and intense suffering, today I enjoy abundant good health! I have almost unlimited strength and energy, and I work hard each day in a factory. Thanks to the raw juices I am now completely without pain. (See illustration on page 104.)

––––––––––––––– ◇ –––––––––––––––

Science reveals the cause of illness, and, in a large measure, how to prevent it. YOUR FOOD DETERMINES IN A LARGE MEASURE HOW LONG YOU SHALL LIVE — how much you shall enjoy life, and how successful your life shall be.

CHAPTER EIGHT

"IF THE DOCTOR OF TODAY DOES
NOT BECOME THE DIETICIAN OF
TOMORROW, THE DIETICIAN OF
TODAY WILL BECOME THE DOCTOR
OF TOMORROW."

— Dr. Alexis Carrel,
Rockefeller Institute of Medical Research.

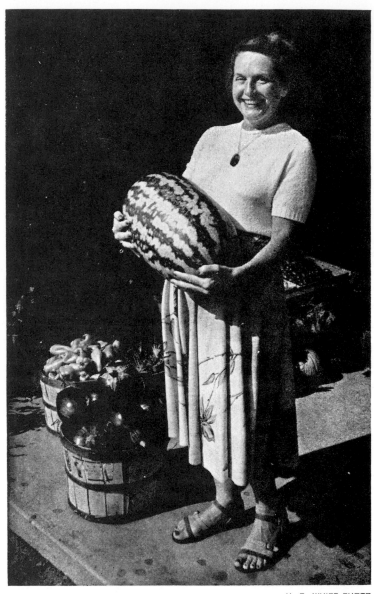

A happy customer struggles with a 30-pound monster from Phil Arena's famous organic watermelon patch, near Escondido, California.

Essential Minerals For Body Building

CERTAIN organic minerals compose the structure of the cells of our bodies, and unless they are made available in our daily foods the cells are starved. Ill health and eventual death results. From U.S. Senate Document No. 264, I quote:

"It is bad news to learn from leading authorities that 99% of the American people are deficient in these minerals, and that a marked deficiency in any one of the more important minerals actually *results in disease.* Any upset of the balance, any considerable lack of one or another element, however microscopic the body requirement may be, and we sicken, suffer, shorten our lives."

What are these minerals that form the essential materials from which this building we call the body is composed? This chapter will be devoted to a presentation of the most vital of these minerals, and briefly describe the function of each in the human body.

PHOSPHORUS

Phosphorus is an essential constituent of every cell in the body, but ninety per cent of it is found in the bony structure. It is also widely distributed in the soft tissues and body fluids. Total amounts are not large, but they must be supplied daily for health.

CALCIUM

There is a considerable difference between the amounts of calcium required for life, and that required for buoyant health. Calcium has recently been recognized as having a far larger and far reaching effect than previously believed. It is now known to aid better growth — a longer period of healthy middle life — extension of life expectancy, and the postponement of senility. With women, when calcium was increased, their children became more healthy and the mother enjoyed better health and longer life. A deficiency is in evidence when an expectant mother loses her teeth during pregnancy. Nature's demands for the infant will not be denied. The mother suffers tragic loss because of the lack of calcium.

CHLORINE

An antiseptic factor in the system.

COPPER

Scientists tell us that while copper does not enter directly in the constitution of the hemoglobin molecule, it does exercise an essential influence. Shortage of copper holds up the process of building the hemoglobin. While other factors may enter into producing anemia, in a very real sense the cause is nutritional.

IRON

Iron is the nucleus of every cell. It is the outstanding material in the red blood cells. It has the important task of carrying oxygen through the system. Shortage of iron means anemia. Iron in human nutrition is involved with the formation and regeneration in the building of the red cells of the blood. It is the cure and prevention of anemia (other than in cases of pernicious anemia, which scientists tell us comes from a gastric juice deficiency). Iron is the essential element in the building and upkeep of the blood, a very complex process.

MAGNESIUM

"Magnesium is a very important ingredient in chlorophyll, the green coloring matter in plants. If the magnesium content of the diet is reduced to a very low level, a little less than two parts per million of the diet, experimental animals become sick and die. The blood vessels expand, the heart beats more rapidly, the animals become irritable and finally die in convulsions. There is evidence that in some way magnesium aids in the assimilation of fat in the diet." — U. S. Yearbook of Agriculture.

MANGANESE

Manganese deficiency results in poor bone formation, drowsiness, and a tendency toward apoplexy.

POTASSIUM

Potassium is very prominent both in the blood cells and the soft tissues of the body, and is therefore, a nutritional necessity.

SILICON

Silicon deficiency results in a tendency toward neuritis, scaly and scabby skin.

SODIUM

Valuable in balancing fluids in the tissues.

IODINE

Goitre is the sign of a lack of iodine in the system. Goitre is caused by an abnormal enlargement of the cells when nature attempts to produce sufficient iodine. Iodine is utilized to produce thyroid hormones necessary for physical and mental well-being. The vegetables in the California area are rich sources of iodine. The ample use of the same is a good defense against goitre.

Daily Requirement Small

The daily requirement of the body is small but the regular health-demands for organic minerals is persistent and perpetual. To ignore that demand is to invite illness. If we can visualize the cells of our bodies as building blocks, and the minerals as essential ingredients of every block, we can readily understand how necessary it is that we have foods rich in these essentials.

In the December, 1945 Reader's Digest there appeared an article of startling significance, entitled: "Are We Starving To Death?" In this article an eminent "Soil Doctor," Wm. A. Albrecht, Ph.D., chairman of the Department of Soils, University of Missouri, warns us:

"Doctors through experiment and observation, began to understand that many diseases could be traced to dietary deficiencies, and that many sick people were hungry people. They called it 'hidden hunger' because people might eat three square meals a day and still suffer from it.

"One of the 'hidden hungers' was for calcium a shortage of which could cause rickets. Goitre was hooked up with a shortage of iodine; night blindness with a shortage of carotene; anemia with iron and possibly copper shortage; thyroid troubles with a shortage of zinc; tooth decay with shortages of calcium phosphorus and fluorine.

"Nations or individuals, men or animals, *we are what we eat.* . . . A properly mineral-rich diet predisposes a man to health and normal functioning, and the healthier we are, the better we resist disease."

To demonstrate this in plants, Dr. Albrecht took the writer of this article into a greenhouse where several varieties of spinach were being fed on different diets, ranging from mineral-rich to mineral-poor. Thrips had nearly destroyed the poorly-fed spinach plants, but not one of the richly-fed plants showed a sign of attack. They had something that enabled them to resist. "In the same way," Albrecht said, "people who have the proper elements in their diets are more resistant to certain diseases."

CHAPTER NINE

"IT IS THROUGH IGNORANCE
THAT THE COMMUNITY IS SUR-
FEITED WITH UNSUITABLE FOODS
. . . PEOPLE WHO EAT NATURAL
FOODS NEVER EAT TOO MUCH."
— *Dr. Bircher-Benner.*

	BEET (Red)	CARROT	CELERY	CUCUMBER	Romaine LETTUCE	PARSLEY	RHUBARB	
PROTEIN %	1.6	1.1	1.1	0.8	1.2	3.5	0.6	2.
FAT %	0.1	0.4	0.1	0.2	0.3	1.0	0.7	0.
CARBOHYDRATE %	9.7	9.3	3.3	3.1	3.0	9.0	3.8	3.
CALORIES PER PINT	220	217	89	84	94	283	115	1
CALCIUM %	0.140	0.225	0.390	0.050	0.345	0.350	0.220	0.
MAGNESIUM %	1.130	0.100	0.140	0.045	0.065	0.160	0.085	0
POTASSIUM %	1.770	1.540	1.460	0.700	1.660	1.50	1.625	2
SODIUM %	0.485	0.385	0.645	0.050	0.100	0.200	0.125	0.
PHOSPHORUS %	0.210	0.205	0.230	0.105	0.140	0.130	0.090	0
CHLORINE %	0.290	0.195	0.665	0.150	0.395	0.090	0.180	0.
SULPHUR %	0.090	0.110	0.140	0 155	0.130	0.120	0.065	0.
IRON %	0.004	0.003	0.003	0.002	0.007	0.016	0.003	0
SILICON %	0.009	0.007	0.008	0.013	0.018		0.006	0.
MANGANESE %	0.008	0.0005	0.0014	0.0013	0.0064	0.008	0.0013	0
COPPER %	0.001	0.007	0.001	0.016	0.0003	0.015	0.0005	0.
IODINE % Parts per billion.	230	180		500	650			4

Oxalic Acid is a relatively prominent factor in Rhubarb, Beet, Chard and other vegetables of so-called goosefoot family.

IMPORTANT JUICES

U. S. Dept. of Agriculture Chart

	WATERCRESS	APPLE	COCONUT	GRAPE	GRAPEFRUIT	LEMON	ORANGE	PINEAPPLE	POMEGRANATE
9	1.7	0.1	1.4	1.3	0.4	0.9	0.6	0.4	1.5
4	0.3	0.2	12.5	1.6	0.1	0.6	0.1	0.3	1.6
0	3.3	12.5	7.0	19.2	9.8	8.7	13.0	9.7	19.5
2	109	250	700	462	200	210	265	207	472
055	0.785	0.035	0.120	0.055	0.105	0.110	0.120	0.040	0.030
065	0.170	0.040	0.100	0.045	0.045	0.045	0.055	0.050	0.020
335	1.435	0.640	1.500	0.530	0.805	0.615	0.905	1.350	1.600
060	0.495	0.055	0.180	0.025	0.020	0.030	0.060	0.080	0.250
145	0.230	0.060	0.370	0.050	0.100	0.055	0.090	0.055	0.050
145	0.305	0.025	0.600	0.010	0.025	0.030	0.025	0.255	0.068
070	0.835	0.030	0.140	0.045	0.050	0.045	0.050	0.045	0.040
002	0.015	0.002		0.0015	0.0014	0.003	0.002	0.002	0.004
009		0.006		0.002			0.0007		
0012	0.0036	0.0003	0.0017	0.0001	0.0001	0.0002	0.0003	0.006	
0005	0.005	0.0008	0.0009	0.0005	0.0003		0.0008	0.0004	0.0005
50	180							200	120

Chemists advise against use of same where there is evidence of calcium deficiency.

A WORD OF APPRECIATION

FROM AN ILLINOIS READER

Dear Dr. Kirschner:

It was so kind of you to take the time to answer my letter of last year. You asked me to write again some day and tell you how I was coming along.

I follow faithfully the exact diet listed in chapter thirteen of your book. I love it and never touch any other food. The only trouble I ever encounter is when the family goes to a restaurant; but my husband is very careful to have special salads made to order for me. I usually bring my own dressing made from the recipe you gave me.

I still don't weigh too much, but I am amazed at the amount of energy I have for my teaching and writing and caring for my family. And of course, no doctor bills, because we never have to go to one! My family doctor has no idea how "queerly" I eat, but he does know of our drinking fresh vegetable juices, and is delighted with my eleven-year-old daughter's superb health and mental alertness. All three of our children are straight A students in school.

Several of my friends have watched my program of drinking fresh vegetable juices and have bought your book and a juicer too. When anyone asks me who my doctor is, I always say proudly, "Dr. Kirschner."

If you every publish any new material, be sure and let me know. And thank you again for your kindness and marvelous help. It's such fun to be healthy and enjoy life so much!

— Mrs. W. R. Augsburger.

Vitamins and
Their Sources

WHAT ARE VITAMINS? The chemist tells us they are small quantities of substances essential to life. They are found in every living structure. For the most part in green growing plants on land and in algae and other organisms in the sea. Many of these substances have been isolated chemically and we have names for them. A, B, C, D, E, etc. But there are unquestionably others not yet discovered or isolated, that are just as necessary for the maintenance of life. That is the reason scientists give for the use of *natural foods,* such as vegetables, to combat malnutrition, instead of using a synthetic chemical, although they may be identical in essence. Doctor Borsook tells of patients suffering from a severe deficiency of Vitamin A (the anti-infection vitamin). When huge doses of the synthetic vitamin were given, the patients' condition did not improve; but when FOOD containing all the vitamins was given, there was rapid recovery. His concluding statement was: "Vitamins worked better in concert with all other vitamins." The complete vitamin complex is found only in NATURE. It never has, and never will come from a test-tube in some laboratory!

VITAMIN A

Vitamin A combats infection. Lack of it results in retarded growth, impaired teeth, eyes and bones; the shortening of the life span; blindness in the glare of light; impaired vision in dim light. Vitamin A deficiency also results in many skin diseases, cirrhosis of the liver, kidney stones; also degeneration of nerve fibres.

VITAMIN B
Vitamin B represents a whole family of vitamins called the "B Complex." Deficiency symptoms include: A lack of appetite, neuritis, constipation, excessive fat, heart disease, enlargement of the heart, arthritis, and poor metalobism of starches and sugars.

VITAMIN C
Deficiency symptoms include scurvy (evidenced in subnormal growth), lowered resistance to infection, paleness, discoloring of the skin, rapid pulse, hemorrhage of gums, anemia, teeth that loosen and fall out.

VITAMIN D
Vitamin D is called the Sunshine vitamin. It is a cure for rickets. Rickets is a disease of the growing parts of the bone in which the normal amounts of calcium and phosphorus are deposited. The system is unable to use calcium and phosphorus in the building of bone without an adequate supply of Vitamin D. Vitamin D may be obtained from fish liver oils, from green plants, and from sun bathing.

VITAMIN E
Vitamin E is known as the "anti-sterility" vitamin. The chief source is from green vegetables and wheat germ oil. This important vitamin prevents miscarriage. Some clinics have used it in the treatment of heart disease. A deficiency of Vitamin E often leads to degeneration of the skeotal muscles.

VITAMIN K
Vitamin K enables the blood to coagulate. It is, therefore, the anti-hemorrhage vitamin. It also assists in the normal function of the liver. This vitamin is often used by surgeons a few days before an operation. It also reduces the death rate from hemorrhage in the case of new-born babies.

SOME OF THE BEST SOURCES OF MINERALS AND VITAMINS

In the preceding chapter we have talked about minerals and their vital role in the maintenance of a healthy, vibrant-with-life body structure. In our present chapter we are discussing the mysterious and all-important entities called VITAMINS. What are the best sources of these essential elements? We present herewith a partial list of fruits and vegetables that are richest in nutritive value, and which can be taken conveniently in the form of juice.

APPLE JUICE

Apple juice is rich in magnesium, iron and silicon. It also contains potassium, a valuable aid to digestion, plus phosphorus, sodium, calcium, sulphur and chlorine. Malic acid, reputed to be a cleansing agent and healer of internal inflammation, is found in apple juice. Its vitamins include A, B, C and G.

BEET JUICE

Beet juice contains an abundance of sodium (over 50%). It also contains iron, calcium, potassium, and chlorine. It is considered one of the most valuable juices for the liver and gall bladder, and for building up the red corpuscles, and stimulates the activity of the lymph throughout the entire body. It contains Vitamins A, B, C and G.

CUCUMBER JUICE

Cucumbers are a medium source of Vitamins A and B, and are a rich source of Vitamin C. Cucumbers are usually ruined nutritionally by the addition of salt and vinegar. They are very rich in potassium, iron and magnesium. They also rate high in silicon and chlorine, and are considered by scientists as a top-flight health vegetable.

CABBAGE JUICE

This popular vegetable contains chlorine, calcium, sodium and iron. It is rich in Vitamins A, B, C, G and U. Dr. Chaney of the Stanford Medical School reveals that Vitamin U in cabbage juice is a very important factor in healing stomach ulcers, both duodenal and peptic.

CARROT JUICE

Carrots are exceedingly rich in Vitamin A (medium source of B, C, and G). In recent years carrots have been recognized as one of the most valuable of vegetables. Carrot juice is very delicious, and it is perhaps the best balanced vegetable from the standpoint of both minerals and vitamins. Scientists tell us that the iron and calcium of carrots is almost entirely assimilable. Raw carrots contain nearly all the minerals and vitamins that are required by the human body. Carotene is the vegetable form of Vitamin A. It also contains the mineral content of potassium, iron, magnesium, manganese, sodium, silicon and iodine. In addition it contains the strong cleansing elements of sulphur, chlorine, and phosphorus. Dr. Sherman states that carrots are one of the best sources of calcium, which is a crucial element in the maintenance of optimal health.

CELERY JUICE

Celery is very high in sodium, magnesium and iron. It also contains liberal quantities of potassium, calcium, sulphur, and magnesium. It is an excellent source of Vitamins A, B, C, and E. Celery has become famous as a nerve tonic, and aids in the elimination of carbon dioxide from the system.

COCOANUT JUICE

Cocoanuts are rich in potassium, chlorine, phosphorus, sodium, sulphur, calcium, magnesium and iron. They contain Vitamins A, B, and G. The high Vitamin B content aids in digestive disturbances.

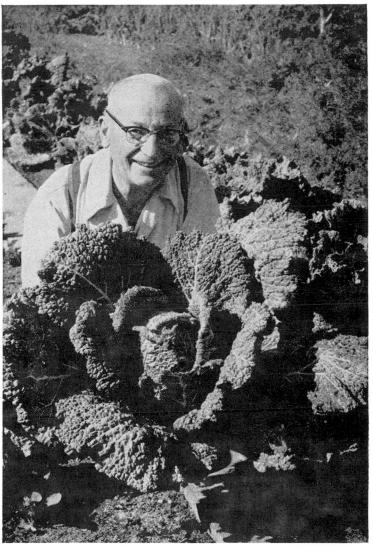

The author proudly displays one of his giant home-grown cabbages — rich in Vitamins C and U, and other essential minerals and vitamins.

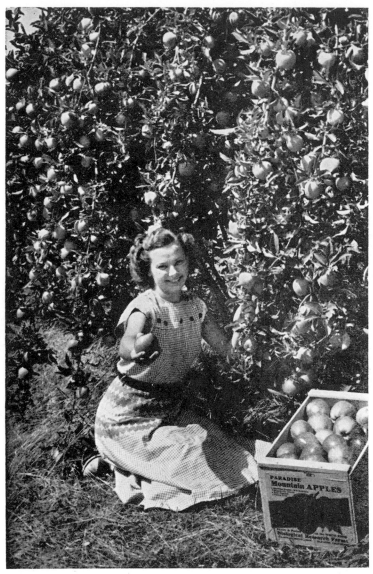

Our attractive young "Miss" from Paradise is following in the footprints of her ancestor — "Mother Eve" — as she temptingly holds out one of Herbert White's delicious, organically-grown apples on his 10-acre Paradise (California) fruit farm.

DANDELION JUICE

Dandelion is highly regarded as a source of vital organic magnesium. It also contains potassium, sodium, chlorine, calcium, phosphorus, sulphur, silicon and iron. Dandelion juice is considered one of our most valuable tonics. It gives strength and firmness to the teeth, preventing pyorrhea and decay. It is a good source of Vitamins A, B, C and G.

ENDIVE JUICE

Endive is closely related to the Dandelion family, and its constituents are more or less alike. It is rich in potassium, magnesium, chlorine, sodium, calcium, phosphorus, sulphur and iron. Endive is one of the finest sources of Vitamin A. It also contains Vitamins C and G. It also is bitter, and should be blended with carrot and celery juice.

KALE JUICE

Kale is regarded as an outstanding source of Vitamin A. During the war it became important in maintaining excellent health conditions in Britain in spite of severe rationing. It is rich in calcium and riboflavin — a B Vitamin. Kale is also rich in iron, phosphorus, sulphur and potassium. A cup of Kale leaves contains 37,000 units of Vitamin A, and 2,900 units of Vitamin C.

LEMON JUICE

Lemons are the richest foods on earth in bio-flavonoids; and bio-flavonoids play a dramatic role in our search for health and longevity. They not only help to regulate the body chemistry, but they are unsurpassed in influencing the life processes. Lemons are very rich in Vitamin C, and produce spectacular results in relieving the common cold.

LETTUCE JUICE

Lettuce has an abundance of potassium, sodium, calcium, phosphorus and iodine. It is particularly rich in magnesium and iron. One of the most nourishing of foods for the cells and tissues of the nervous and muscular structures of the body. Its vitamins include A, B, C, E and G. The green leafy lettuce is best, as it contains more of the life-giving chlorophyll. It, too, is bitter, and should be used in combination with carrot and celery juice.

ONION JUICE

Onions are a moderate source of Vitamins A, B and G. They are an excellent source of C. They rate high in antiseptic qualities. Onions are abundant in minerals, including potassium, sulphur, phosphorus, calcium, chlorine, magnesium, iron and iodine. Scientists tell us that onions aid digestion. As the juice has a very strong flavor, it should be used in combination with the milder juices.

PARSLEY JUICE

Parsley juice is said to be one of the most potent of vegetable juices. It should, therefore, be taken in small quantities (one or two ounces), blended with carrot, celery or lettuce juice. Parsley is rich in potassium, calcium, sodium, magnesium, phosphorus, sulphur, chlorine and iron. It is a good source of Vitamins A, B, C and E. Parsley aids in oxygen metabolism, and helps in maintaining normal action of the adrenal and thyroid glands.

PEA POD JUICE

When fresh pea pods are juiced, an ingredient is obtained that aids the pancreas in its function.

PINEAPPLE JUICE

Pineapple is especially rich in essential minerals — potassium, chlorine, sodium, phosphorus, magnesium, sulphur, calcium, iron and iodine. It also contains the ferment Bromelin, which parallels the pancreatic secretion. Its Vitamins are A, B, C and G. It is one of our most delicious and healthgiving juices when eaten raw and unsweetened.

RADISH JUICE

According to nutritional authorities nearly one-third of the content of radishes is potassium. Another one-third is sodium. The iron and magnesium content are also high. Other minerals include sulphur, chlorine, phosphorus, calcium and iodine. Its vitamins are A, B, and C. It has a soothing and healing effect on the mucous membranes of the body.

SPINACH JUICE

According to Dr. N. W. Walker, "In raw spinach, Nature has furnished man with the finest organic material for the cleansing, reconstruction and regeneration of the intestinal tract." Spinach is a good source of potassium, sodium, calcium, iodine, magnesium, phosphorus, sulphur and iron. It contains liberal quantities of Vitamins A, B, C, E and G.

TOMATO JUICE

Tomato juice is rich in magnesium, iron, potassium, phosphorus, chlorine, sulphur, calcium, sodium and iodine. Tomatoes are also rich in vegetable amino acids. They are an excellent source of Vitamin C, and contain others, such as A, B, and G.

TURNIP TOP JUICE

When juiced, turnip tops are valuable as a source of iron, calcium, potassium, chlorine, sodium, sulphur, phosphorus, and magnesium. They contain Vitamins A, B, C, E and G. Turnip tops are about three times as rich as orange or tomato juice in Vitamin C.

WATERCRESS JUICE

Watercress is rich in potassium, sulphur, calcium, sodium, chlorine, phosphorus, magnesium, iron and iodine. Scientists tell us that one-third of the mineral content of watercress is sulphur, and that 45% of the elements are acid forming. It should, therefore, never be taken alone, but in combination with carrot and celery juices. It is a powerful intestinal cleanser, and also assists in the normal regeneration of the blood. Its Vitamins include A, B, C, E and G.

POTATO JUICE

The juice of raw potatoes is high in potassium, sulphur, phosphorus and chlorine, and thus has proved very beneficial in clearing up skin blemishes. This cleansing action is present *only* in the *raw* potato where the live organic atoms can perform their beneficent task. As the potato juice is not very palatable when taken alone, it can be combined with that of other vegetable juices.

GREEN PEPPER JUICE

Green pepper juice is rich in silicon, and therefore, is beneficial to the nails and hair. It also helps in clearing up skin blemishes, flatulence and colic. It combines nicely with carrot juice — 25% green pepper with 75% carrot.

STRAWBERRY JUICE

Strawberry juice is one of the most useful as well as the most appetizing of juices. It contains much fruit sugar and iron, making it valuable as an aid to a good complexion. In fact it is one of the best skin cleansers known. It should be taken regularly in cases of poor complexion, anemia, skin eruption, sluggish liver, constipation, acidosis and catarrh. It has proved to be a good tonic for glands and nerves.

ORANGE JUICE

The value of orange juice is widely recognized today. As a dietary supplement for infants and growing children it stands high on the list because of its power to assist in bone formation, and in preventing rickets. Orange juice is high in fruit sugar, and is a source of calcium and phosphorus. It is valuable as a blood cleanser.

CHAPTER TEN

"THE FACT IS THERE IS ONLY
ONE MAJOR DISEASE, AND THAT IS
MALNUTRITION. ALL AILMENTS
AND AFFLICTIONS TO WHICH WE
MAY BECOME HEIRS ARE DIRECTLY
TRACEABLE TO THIS MAJOR DIS-
EASE."

— *Dr. C. W. Cavanaugh, Cornell University.*

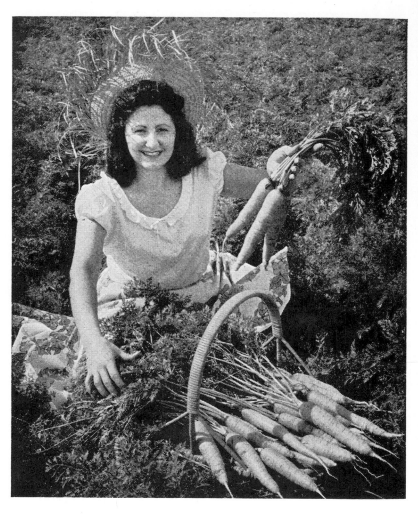

H. C. WHITE PHOTO

Here in the basket are enough freshly-dug carrots to make one gallon of pure, fresh carrot juice. The young lady out in the carrot patch — holding up a bunch of these golden beauties — is none other than the daughter of "Mrs. X" — the famous "carrot juice woman."

Recommendations for Use of Raw Juices

EVER SINCE the first two editions of LIVE FOOD JUICES came off the press, I have received an avalanche of inquiries from readers far and near asking "How much of the live food juices should I take daily in order to relieve my particular ailment or condition?"

The answer to the above question is not as easy as it may seem, for it is always difficult for a doctor or dietitian to prescribe definite amounts of the various juices for the relief of specific ailments without a first-hand knowledge of the patient's condition. However, there are certain general principles that guide us as we seek an answer to our problem.

It is well to remember that in any disease that involves tissue degeneration, our goal is not to palliate certain distressing symptoms, but the rejuvenation and reconstruction of the entire being. The bloodstream must be cleansed, and the defective "building-blocks" must be replaced by those that are sound and in perfect mineral balance.

You may recall the statement made by Dr. Henry Sherman on page 20 of this volume. Here the world's greatest authority on the subject of foods states: "When nutritional knowledge is sufficiently widespread, people will consume up to three pounds of green and yellow vegetables and fruits daily." Roughly, three pounds of whole vegetables or fruits will make a pound and one-half of raw juices, or the equivalent of one and one-half pints.

The above statement by one of America's most noted authorities, gives us a "clue" on which to base the proper daily intake of these live food juices. Certain conditions, however, may make it necessary to use much less of the juices at first, during the more critical stage of the illness; increasing the amount as the patient's condition improves.

In the case of Mrs. X, you will recall, her condition was so desperate when she first started the raw juice therapy, it was necessary for her to take the carrot juice by the spoonful. Gradually, as her condition improved, the amount was increased to an 8-ounce glass daily. Finally, she was able to take one gallon of juice per day. No other food was allowed during her recovery period, which accounts for the very large amount of juice required in her daily regimen.

In the case of Mr. B, who suffered from cancer of the bladder and kidney; at the first he drank only one glassful of carrot juice (6-8 ounces) a day. Later he increased the amount to two quarts per day, until his recovery was complete. The late Dr. Max Gerson, former cancer specialist of New York City required his patients to take a minimum of thirty-two ounces of live food juices daily — mostly in the form of carrot and apple.

Some dietitians recommend a minimum of sixteen ounces of the fruit and vegetable juices per day. Various combinations include carrot, celery, beet, parsley, spinach, cucumber, apple, grape, pineapple, cocoanut, etc. But in every *combination* carrot juice predominates (8-12 ounces); Spinach, 2-8 ounces; Celery, 4-8 ounces; Beet, 2-5 ounces; Cucumber, 3-5 ounces; Parsley, 2-4 ounces; Apple, 8 ounces; Orange, 8 ounces; Grapefruit, 8 ounces; Watercress, 8 ounces; Pineapple, 8 ounces; Coconut, 4 ounces.

The following is a list of common ailments that we believe will respond most favorably to raw juice therapy. Remember, our aim is to cleanse the bloodstream, and thus build the body's fighting mechanism, and to relieve the CAUSE of these painful disorders. In each case, the formulas should be prepared from pure raw fruit and vegetable juices — fresh from the juicer, and if possible the produce used should be organically grown, free from toxic insecticides.

1. ACNE (Skin disorders) — Carrot, lettuce, spinach, beet, cucumber, grape, apricot, green pepper, raw potato.
2. ALLERGIES — Carrot, celery, beet, cucumber.
3. ANEMIA — Carrot, beet, celery, **spinach, parsley,** watercress.
4. ANGINA PECTORIS — Carrot, celery, spinach.
5. ARTHRITIS — Carrots, **celery,** beet, cucumber.
6. ASTHMA — Carrot, spinach, celery.
7. BILIOUSNESS — Carrot, spinach, beet, cucumber, celery, parsley.
8. BLADDER DISEASE — Carrot, celery, spinach, **parsley,** cucumber, beet.
9. BOILS, CARBUNCLES — Carrot, spinach, beet, cucumber.
10. BRONCHITIS — Carrot, spinach, celery, beet, cucumber.
11. CANCER — Carrot, celery, spinach, cabbage, apple.
12. CATARRH — Carrot, celery, spinach, beet, cucumber.
13. COLDS — Carrot, celery, lemon, orange, grapefruit.
14. COLITIS — Carrot, apple, beet, cucumber.
15. CONSTIPATION — Carrot, apple, celery, **spinach,** grape.
16. DERMATITIS — Carrot, celery, apple, beet, cucumber.
17. DIARRHEA — Carrot, **apple,** celery, spinach, parsley, **raspberry, blackberry.**
18. EYE DISEASES (Due to Vitamin Deficiency) — Carrot, spinach, celery, parsley.
19. GOUT — Carrot, celery, spinach, parsley, beet, cucumber.
20. HALITOSIS (Bad Breath) — Carrot, celery, spinach, cucumber.
21. HAY FEVER — Carrot, celery, beet, cucumber, spinach, parsley.
22. HEADACHE — Carrot, spinach, celery, parsley, beet, cucumber, lettuce.
23. HEART TROUBLE (Functional) — Carrot, spinach, celery, parsley, cucumber.
24. HIGH BLOOD PRESSURE — Carrot, cucumber, parsley, spinach, celery, beet.
25. INFLUENZA — Carrot, celery, spinach, beet, cucumber, grapefruit, lemon.
26. INSOMNIA — Carrot, spinach, celery, lettuce.

27. KIDNEY TROUBLE — Juice of ½ lemon in warm water, carrot, dandelion, parsley, spinach, celery, beet, cucumber, grape.

28. LIVER DISORDERS — Carrot, beet, parsley, cucumber, dandelion, radish.

29. MALAISE — Carrot, celery, apple, beet, cucumber, parsley.

30. MIGRAINE (Headache) — Carrot, spinach, celery, parsley.

31. MUCOUS MEMBRANE — Carrot, apple, pineapple, celery, beet, cucumber.

32. NERVE DISORDERS — Lettuce, carrot, celery, apple, spinach, cucumber, beet, radish.

33. OVERWEIGHT — Carrot, celery, spinach, beet, cucumber.

34. PEPTIC ULCER — Cabbage, celery, carrot.

35. PREGNANCY — Carrot, celery, spinach, beet, cucumber, cocoanut, apple, orange.

36. RHEUMATISM — Carrot, celery, spinach, parsley, lettuce, watercress, cucumber.

37. RICKETS — Carrots, celery, spinach, apple, orange, lemon, grapefruit.

38. SCURVY — Carrot, celery, apple, grapefruit, orange, lemon.

39. SINUS TROUBLE — Carrot, spinach, beet, cucumber.

40. TEETH — Carrot, celery, beet, watercress.

41. TONSILITIS — Carrot, celery, pineapple, orange, apple, lemon.

42. TOXEMIA — Carrot, parsley, celery, spinach, cucumber, apple.

43. TUBERCULOSIS — Carrot, alfalfa, parsley, spinach, watercress, comfrey (to be used in green drink).

John B. Lust, well-known nutritionist tells us: "Natural healing is the most desirable factor in the regeneration of the race. It makes use of the elementary forces of Nature, of chemical selection of foods that will constitute a correct medical dietary.

"There is really but one healing force in existence and that is Nature herself: that is the inherent restorative power of the organism to overcome disease. The practical application of these natural agencies, duly suited to the individual case, are the true signs and the whole art of healing. — *Raw Juice Therapy,* page 3.

CHAPTER ELEVEN

A DOG IS MAN'S BEST FRIEND.
MAN IS DOG'S BEST FRIEND!

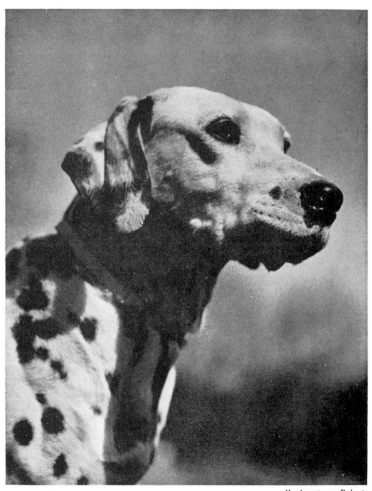

Carrot Juice Therapy Restores Ancient Canine

(A Dog Story)

I HOLD in my hand a most interesting letter from one of my New York readers. In fact, I am so deeply impressed with her story, I have decided to pass it on for the benefit of readers who may encounter a similar problem.

Mr. and Mrs. "S" are the owners of a 12½-year-old Dalmatian of whom they are very proud. These English "Coach Dogs," as they are sometimes called, are highly intelligent, and their habits around the home are usually impeccable.

Unfortunately, a little over one year ago a number of distressing symptoms began to develop which not only upset the orderly routine of the household, but also posed a real threat to the very life of this valuable animal.

Let's have Mrs. "S" tell the story in her own words. Here is her report, dated August 4, 1962.

Dear Dr. Kirschner:

My husband and I are enthusiastic readers and students of your articles and books. We believe you will be interested in our experience with carrot juice administered to our dog.

On August 18, 1961, our veterinarian found that our 11½-year-old Dalmatian had nephritis and a very large abdominal tumor. He prescribed a canned diet to control the urination, which had become excessive and uncontrolled. The doctor said he could do an exploratory operation for the tumor, but did not recommend it in view of the dog's age and other factors. The doctor believed he would find the tumor inoperable and malignant. I returned the dog to the doctor one week later for further examination. He found that the tumor showed further considerable growth, and pronounced it "a very rapid grower." He felt the dog's life expectancy was short.

I gave the dog the prescribed canned diet for four days. By the fifth day his condition deteriorated greatly and he began to lose weight rapidly. He became exceedingly thin and bony. He grew very weak and trembled convulsively for twenty-four hours. During this period, I gave him his first carrot juice, extracted with a centrifugal type juicer. During succeeding days, I increased his carrot juice intake to 32 ounces, then 45 ounces, and finally two quarts daily. Since then, he has taken two quarts of carrot juice daily, almost without exception. During the months when I am able to get unsprayed, organically-grown apples, I also use apples in the juicer. I have occasionally added celery or beets, but he accepts the carrot juice more readily.

I eliminated meat altogether, but he has taken various fruits and vegetables. Within 24 to 36 hours after we had started on the carrot juice, his condition began to improve: his strength began to return and the trembling stopped.

The dog's urination is now completely controlled (a normally fastidious animal, he had previously lost control as often as six times a day in the house). In spite of the high intake of liquids, he has had no problem with his kidneys for many months. He now goes for an eight or nine hour stretch at night without having to get out.

The dog was re-examined monthly for the first few months of his illness, and the doctor found that the tumor was continuing to grow, and had reached the size "the diameter of a grapefruit and about seven inches long." I now have him examined every two months or so, and on the last two visits the doctor said there had been no further growth.

The dog continues to drink two quarts of fresh juice daily, though I now add a few tablespoonfuls of broth (chicken, beef liver, beef kidney, etc.)

In addition to the juices and the fruits and vegetables, etc., he is given a heavy intake of natural vitamins and minerals.

He takes two packages monthly of a well-known food supplement from natural concentrates, and two packages monthly of natural C vitamin tablets. You will note that this is double the amount of each recommended for humans.

The dog regained his lost weight after a few months on the diet. Now, almost one year from the discovery of his tumor and nephritis, he is energetic, clear-eyed and obviously in no pain. He sleeps well and his elimination is normal. The doctor is greatly impressed and says the dog's condition is "marvelous." He attributes it all to the diet, as he is merely examining the patient and not administering treatments.

Sincerely yours,

Mrs. L. E. S.
Flushing, New York

In presenting the above story, no effort is being made to show that carrot juice will ever "cure" a tumor, or any other abnormal growth—malignant or otherwise—in man or dog. But in observing this interesting "case-history" it is obvious that carrot juice DID SOMETHING to that decrepit old Dalmatian that eventually halted the rapid progress of the disease and brought the growth to a standstill as well as restoring normal kidney and bladder function.

"COMMENTARY ON JUICES"

Within recent months certain documents from the Division of Scientific Activities of the American Medical Association have come to my desk. I was much interested to find in one of these a discussion of the nutritional value of vegetable juice—particularly carrot juice.

The author points out that certain manufacturers of juice extractors imply in their advertising that "converting vegetables to juices will, in some manner improve the nutritional value of the final product." Obviously the process of converting vegetables into juice cannot ADD to their mineral, vitamin or enzyme content. The added value lies in the increased amounts of these substances one can consume when the vegetables are in juice form. Therefore, a good juicer is an investment in health.

These facts are emphasized by well-known nutritional authorities, R. D. Pope, M.D., and N. W. Walker, D.Sc. In their book, Raw Vegetable Juices, they state: "to overcome the deficiency of live, organic mineral salts in the human body, an abundant use of raw vegetable juices is essential because the digestive tract cannot assimilate the volume of bulk otherwise required by eating raw vegetables and fruits in sufficient quantities. As it is the chemistry of the individual that makes him what he is, the copious intake of raw vegetable juices will so re-chemicalize the body that nature will take care of the elimination of disease and the regeneration of the cells and the tissues."

This simple, natural, body-building program is proving beneficial to tens of thousands of our readers. Letters come to my desk every day from enthusiastic persons who are faithfully following this program. Following are some examples:

Dear Dr. Kirschner: I am a retired druggist, 64 years of age. I have read your books and most of your articles. I have had rheumatoid arthritis for many years, and until about four months ago was almost totally disabled. On February 1st of this year (1961) I discontinued the use of all cooked foods, and began living on two or three quarts of carrot juice during the day, and a salad or a dish of Museli for dinner at night. This is supplemented with your "Green Drink" whenever any good greens are available.

After about four months of this routine I began to notice some diminution of pain and an increased mobility. *Today, seven months later, I can walk without crutches!* This is something I have not been able to do for years.

P.S.B.   Arizona

Dear Dr. Kirschner: A friend and I became interested in live food juices and last November started on them. I have colitis and the juices have helped me immensely. I was also subject to viruses and infections and have really developed resistance against them because of the carrot juice. My friend has arthritis and has had several operations. We are both waitresses and depend on our hands a lot. Hers swell and give her pain at night and during the day too. She is drinking about a pint of celery juice a day and a quart of carrot juice with greens mixed in such as spinach and endive juice.

We have benefited greatly from your book and can't imagine being without our juices. At this date I have lost seventeen pounds and hope to lose about seven to ten more. It is the first time I haven't gotten sick from dieting. Needless to say my juicer would be the last thing I would part with. I plan to take it with me on my vacation. Most important is my little girl benefits from it. My little girl who is almost nine has had an allergic rhinitis since almost birth and has suffered a lot with viruses and infections. We had occasion to go to the doctor about a month after we started taking juices. Of course the doctor pooh-poohed the idea of juices and said "IT WAS A RACKET." *However, he said her nose was in much better condition and the pus and sores and inflammation gone.* The medicine he gave her was so bad tasting I didn't make her take it after the first day and we haven't been back since or felt the need to. She feels better and I am hoping for a complete cure.

Prior to taking the juices I believe I mentioned that I was barely able to drag myself to work. Well I really accomplish things now and I'm very busy. I am able now to take art lessons, something I've wanted to do for a long time. I am a very nervous person and while I haven't completely overcome that as yet, I don't feel like I am always on tenterhooks as I used to be. I DON'T NEED TRANQUILIZERS ANY MORE AND I USED TO TAKE THEM ALL THE TIME. That alone is worth a lot to me.

Again I want to thank you for giving me a new lease on life.   Mrs. M. E.

Dear Dr. Kirschner: Last September I came down with sciatica and after much suffering and spending three weeks in a hospital—where they discovered I had too much uric acid in my blood—I came home. Then had a relapse with the pain which was very severe. In fact, so bad I was confined to my home for two weeks. This pain settled in my lower back.

I was desperate and willing to try anything. I bought a juicer and started on carrot and celery juices. The results were almost miraculous, for in about a week I was back at work and felt almost as good as I ever did. People who know me and saw me when I was in so much misery cannot believe that it was possible for me to make such a quick recovery. Many thanks for what your information did for me.

                                                Mr. L. J. J.

"IT'S NOT THE FOOD IN YOUR LIFE BUT THE LIFE IN YOUR FOOD THAT COUNTS!"

CHAPTER TWELVE

"MORE LIVES CAN BE SAVED FOR
THE EFFORT EXPENDED, DOLLAR
FOR DOLLAR, BY GETTING THE
VERY *BEST NUTRITION* FOR ALL
OUR PEOPLE THAN WE CAN EVER
GAIN WITH CURATIVE OR PREVEN-
TIVE MEDICINE. . . CREATIVE MEDI-
CINE MUST BE FOUNDED ON GROW-
ING THE BEST FOODS. THUS ALONE
CAN WE CREATE REAL HEALTH
FOR OUR PEOPLE."

— Dr. Jonathan Forman,
President, Friends of the Land.

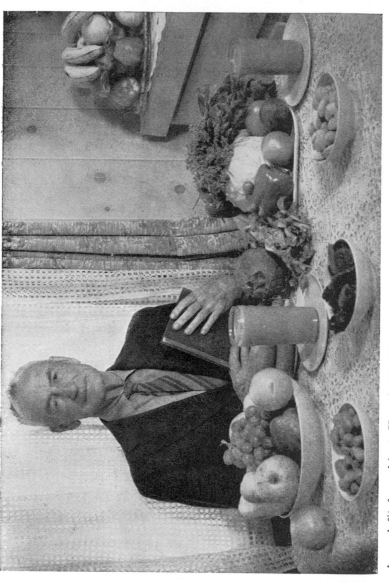

A meal fit for a king! Here is M. Diltz, raw-fooder and devotee of live food juices, ready for his noon-day meal. What a spread of Nature's bounties! Diltz is holding the book "Nature the Healer" by John T. Richter, the book that inspired him to go in for raw-food.

Raw Food Juices Help Restore Failing Eyes

ONE Sunday morning last fall while sitting under the shade of the umbrella tree in my Yucaipa garden, a car drove up to the garden gate, and out stepped a lively old man, who walked to the spot where I was sitting.

"Are you Doctor Kirschner?" he inquired. When I answered in the affirmative, he said: "For a long time I have wanted to meet you, Doctor. I have read and re-read your book *Live Food Juices,* and have followed your program faithfully for over two years. Would you like to hear my story?" Of course I said "Yes," and hereby hangs a tale that I know will be of interest to all my readers.

The following narrative is the result of our conversation that brisk Sunday morning, and reveals the almost miraculous restoration of a sick man to health and activity through simple, natural methods. The experience of this rejuvenated old man of 77 years, emphasizes once again the dictum of Hippocrates, famous Greek physician, who declared: "Leave your drugs in the chemist's pot if you can heal the patient with food!"

My new-found friend, Mr. M. Diltz, was born in Eaton, Ohio, in the year 1883. He moved to California in 1906. For 52 years he operated a one-man barber shop. At the age of 30 young Mr. Diltz began to suffer from varicose veins, and at 49 other uncomfortable and alarming symptoms revealed the fact that all was not well with this busy, enterprising barber. For 12 years he was the unhappy victim of *tic douloureux,* a distressing and excruciatingly painful spasmodic neuralgia of the facial nerve. Relief from this rare ailment came after a surgical operation, in which the fifth cranial nerve was removed. During these

12 years of suffering (1932-1944) Diltz took, on doctor's orders, 18 aspirin tablets per day to relieve the pain.

In 1942, at the age of 59, Diltz's physical troubles were multiplied by a severe attack of diabetes, and in 1954 at the age of 71 he was almost completely incapacitated by yellow jaundice. His poor, overworked liver was finally ready to quit functioning, and so were his eyes. So, in addition to all his other troubles he was faced with the prospect of complete blindness. In fact one oculist informed him that his eyes would only last another 30 days.

It was then that Mr. Diltz woke up. After years of drug medication he at last went to an osteopathic physician for help. This doctor recommended that he try DIET as a means of regaining his lost health. Under the wise care of this physician Diltz eliminated meat and all other animal products from his diet. One day — he calls it a "red-letter" day — he discovered a book called *Nature, the Healer,* by John T. Richter. He also found help for his failing eyes through the Bates Treatment, as outlined in Dr. R. A. Richardson's book, and in spite of his advanced age, his eyesight has miraculously improved.

After so many years of physical suffering, Mr. Diltz and his faithful wife became interested in the *cause* of disease, and they studied many books on the subject of HEALTH. It was a long hard struggle to find and put into practice the SEVEN ESSENTIALS OF HEALTH — (1) Fresh air.   (2) Natural food.   (3) Pure water. (4) Sunshine.   (5) Exercise.   (6) Rest.   (7) Mental attitude.

Their determined search for these "seven essentials" led Mr. and Mrs. Diltz away from the crowded cities and out into the clean air and warm sunshine of the desert. In Twenty-nine Palms, California, he at last found the environment best suited to "rebuild" his broken, pain-racked body, and he sold his business and with his devoted wife settled down in two little cabins in the high desert.

During these years in the desert his health greatly improved, and three years later he moved to the beautiful Yucaipa Valley, another health "mecca," with a climate and soil favorable for growing all kinds of fruits, nuts, and vegetables.

And there's where you will find Mr. and Mrs. Diltz today — working in the orchard and garden — enjoying to the full the fruits of their labors, and reveling in Nature's precious gift — unspoiled by processing and cooking.

Mr. and Mrs. Diltz agree with Dr. Richter, who suggests that "the human animal once ate all his food fresh from Nature's hands." They bemoan the fact that we in our ultra-modern civilization "have departed from the simplicity of natural foods, and have built up a bewilderingly complex system of feeding our bodies, until it would take a Philadelphia lawyer or an expert cook to tell just how many mixtures go into each of the dishes that appear upon our tables in the guise of daily bread."

In the thought-provoking introduction to her *Cookless Book* Mrs. Vera Richter goes still further in her peroration against the evils of modern cooking. She declares:

"The preparation of a meal takes many hours of exacting toil in a heated temperature and the wearied housewife sees the product of a morning's work vanish in half an hour. If she wonders what is the *use* of it all, her answer is: Chiefly to create painful disturbances in the interior departments of the various members of her family, and to invite consequent doctor's bills and more inefficiency in the individual victims of her cooked foods."

It was not until my visit to the world-famous Bircher-Benner Sanatorium in Zurich, Switzerland, five years ago that I became fully convinced in my own mind regarding the superlative benefits to be found in the meatless, raw-food diet. After witnessing first-hand the many remarkable cures and almost unbelievable case histories of that institution, I can agree with Mrs. Richter's summation of this vital topic as follows:

"After centuries of baking, boiling, and stewing, it is somewhat of a shock to be confronted with the idea of eating one's food unfired. A little thought will convince one, however, that the most delicious part of any meal now served is the *uncooked part.* What about the salads, the delicious vegetable combinations, the melons, berries, avocados, fruit — in short, a growing number of uncooked foods are already being served on the up-to-date table? The idea is rather inviting after all. Of course, NO COOKING would eliminate flesh foods, but there is hardly any argument left for them, anyway, except that perverted appetites still call for a species of cannibalism. The strongest members of the animal kingdom, as well as those with the best dispositions, are nature food eaters."

Our illustration shows Mr. Diltz now 77 years *young,* surrounded by a bounteous supply of the natural foods he has learned to love. In addition to the raw fruits, vegetables, and nuts, he takes a quart of the therapeutic "Green Drink" daily — plus a liberal quantity of freshly prepared carrot and celery juice. In bringing this chapter to a close, let me add four little one-syllable words: Well done, Mr. Diltz!

TWO CLASSES OF FOODS

"There are two classes of foods. Natural and unnatural or 'processed.' The *natural foods* are the only foods which will encourage life — promote strength and endurance, and help restore lost health. The unnatural foods will always interfere with the normal functions of the body, and sooner or later cause disease and decay of the body. You will find the natural foods close to Nature — in the gardens, orchards and fields, tapping all the vital substances from the rain, soil, atmosphere and sunshine — combining these life-giving elements so that they will be exactly right for your digestive system."

— *Seven Essentials of Health, by Dr. Philip Welsh.*

CHAPTER THIRTEEN

"FOOD ALONE CURES MANY DISEASES."

— *Hu Se-Hui,*
Chinese Imperial Physician, 1314 A.D.

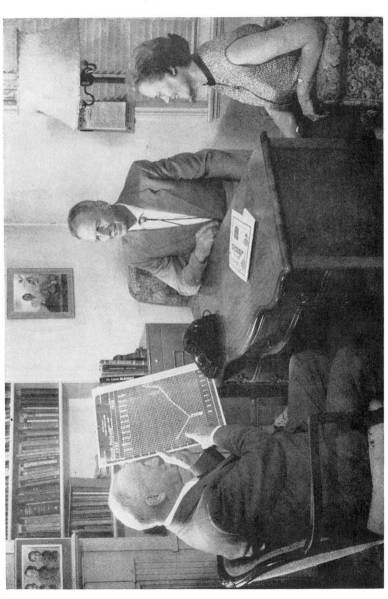

When three raw-fooders get together, there is plenty to talk about! Here the author is shown with Frank and Emma Jean Winkler, from Joliet, Illinois. They had read his book

Papilloma Victim Given One Year to Live!

TEN YEARS ago Frank P. Winkler was a jolly good fellow, who, like the majority of his fellow Americans — *loved to eat.* In fact, when not busy with his prosperous laundry business, he was out searching for new gastronomic thrills. Often this connoisseur of "good food," accompanied by his pretty wife, would drive 150 miles to a famous restaurant for an especially delicious and luscious steak — 300 miles of tortuous driving just for one titallating thrill!

Of course the big steak that Frank loved so much was just one item on the long intriguing menu. Next to a juicy steak *pie* was "Winkler's weakness." In fact, he was just mad about pie — and ice cream! According to the record, in addition, to a score of other rich foods, he and his wife would consume a full quart of ice cream a day. Also for the record, he was a heavy cigar smoker.

Slowly but inexorably all this abundant living had its cumulative effect. Every single ounce of Frank Winkler's high caloric diet seemed to show up on his massive 215-pound frame. Was Winkler concerned about his precarious predicament? Not he! And his neighbors thought the big waistline was becoming indeed — the mark of a prosperous, successful, middle-aged business man.

In 1952, at the age of 54, in addition to the problems concomitant with overweight, other telltale signs and warning signals began to appear in the life of this busy executive. Winkler had long suffered the inconveniences of chronic constipation and bleeding hemorrhoids. In fact from childhood these difficulties had been an integral part of his life pattern. All through the years, he had used laxatives and purgatives in abundance to help Mother Nature in her efforts to "clean house." But these harsh laxatives, including mineral oil, were not the answer to his problem. Year by year, the symptoms became progressively worse.

Another distressing symptom was the increased frequency of urinary evacuations which made it necessary for him to get up many times each night.

Strange as it may seem, neither he nor his wife — nor his doctors — had connected his bad dietetic habits with these unfortunate and unhappy malfunctions of the "body temple." And at least, after decades of abuse, Frank Winkler's big overstuffed body was brought to the point of *no return*. A complete physical collapse was imminent.

The first alarming *acute* symptoms were accompanied by a dangerously high fever of 104 degrees F. He was rushed to a local hospital bed. There he lay for six long weeks in pain so terrible that he was kept in sedation most of the time.

Unable to diagnose his severe illness the local physicians decided to send him to a world-famous clinic for help. At this clinic he was examined by five specialists and underwent exhaustive medical tests to determine the nature and cause of his increasing physical disabilities.

As a result of the tests, it was found that Frank Winkler was a victim of *Papilloma,* or bladder tumors. These wart-like, nipple-shaped growths were so numerous they had greatly reduced the capacity of the bladder to retain urine and had almost blocked the urethra, through which the urine is passed out of the body.

Two of the clinic's physicians advised an immediate operation. The other three specialists did not feel, however, that major surgery was indicated at that time. It was finally decided to perform a trans-urethra resection and cut off these tumors without going through the abdominal wall.

According to Frank Winkler's report, these surgeons did not use the usual cautery treatment, and the consequent bleeding was both profuse and alarming. To ameliorate the terrible hemorrhaging, he was put into a

Sitz bath with alternating hot and cold water. Fortunately, he survived this harrowing ordeal.

The above treatment for the bladder tumors was regarded by the clinic's leading physicians as merely a "temporary measure." Frank and his wife were told in no uncertain terms that unless he submitted to a major operation *soon*, he had *only one year to live*. A few weeks later, the Winklers returned to their home in Joliet, Illinois. And the prospects ahead were anything but rosy.

After this painful and frightening experience at the hospital and clinic, Winkler finally decided to go on a reducing diet. He figured that if he was going to submit to major surgery, his chances for survival were *better* if he slimmed down a bit and got rid of some of the superfluous fat. So, tough as it was for this food-loving gourmet to restrict his eating habits, his desire for survival finally overcame his appetite for rich foods and forced him to reduce the daily intake of calories.

In due time he was rewarded for all his efforts by exhibiting a much reduced waistline. But much to his disappointment and that of his wife, the distressing symptoms noted above still remained a plague him.

It was during one of his yearly vacation trips to Mexico City that Frank became acquainted with a famous Mexican doctor who had "done wonders" in treating the prostate gland. This noted physician sent him to a hospital for X-rays and a cystoscopic examination. The examination showed that numerous *Papilloma* were still clogging the bladder and the urethra. The doctor wanted to perform an immediate operation.

But Frank Winkler had made up his mind about operations. He told that doctor that he would rather *die* than submit to major surgery. So he left Mexico *without* the operation and in the same state of ill health that had brought him there.

On their homeward journey the Winklers stopped off for a few days in Tucson Arizona. Here they found a health food store where they could obtain freshly-pressed carrot juice. On one of their frequent visits to this store, the proprietor offered to demonstrate the juicer for them. He then turned to his book rack where health books were on display, took down a little green book and started to read to them. He read that by taking carrot and parsley juice, made with this machine, Mr. Winkler's serious chronic condition might be relieved. The name of the book was *"Raw Vegetable Juices,"* by Dr. Norman Walker, of Wickenburg, Arizona.

Without further ado, the Winklers purchased a copy of the book, and took it to their motel to read. That night they could not sleep until they had read Dr. Walker's book from cover to cover. Not only were they thrilled with what they read about the magic healing and restorative powers contained in *live food juices,* but they were filled with new hope that at long last they had actually found the way to renewed vitality and lasting *good health.* From their friends at the health food store, they secured Dr. Walker's address and also that of the factory where the juicer was made.

Before leaving their Tucson motel, Mrs. Winkler remarked to her husband, "If we are going to see this scientist (Dr. Walker), we will never be any closer to him than we are right now!"

Frank agreed with his wife, and the following day they headed straight for Wickenburg — Dr. Walker's new headquarters at the Kay-El-Bar Ranch.

On their arrival in Wickenburg, Frank and Emma Jean Winkler made an appointment to see Dr. Walker. From this first interview they received much helpful instruction, and made plans to return to the Kay-El-Bar Health Ranch for a longer stay the following month.

In May, 1957, they spent six weeks studying with Dr. Walker, and according to their enthusiastic report, they enjoyed every minute of it.

On their arrival at the Health Ranch, Mr. Winkler was so weak he could scarcely make his way around without help. However, in less than 10 days on the raw food diet, the live food juices, and with the help of the cleansing colonics and enemas, he regained so much pep and energy that he insisted on mowing the lawns! In fact, he felt like a *new man!*

Early in their stay in Wickenburg the juicer the Winklers had ordered was delivered to them. They were thrilled with their new-found treasure — for they were now equipped to make all their own fresh vegetable juices including parsley and other green, leafy vegetables.

During their six weeks' stay, Dr. Walker discovered that Mr. and Mrs. Winkler were suffering from *worms.* Strange as it may seem, all the X-rays and the meticulous medical examinations made during the years of Frank Winkler's long illness failed to reveal any signs of these health-destroying, voracious and loathsome creatures.

I am glad to report that the high enemas and colonics recommended by Dr. Walker resulted in the eventual passing of 1,510 worm segments from Frank Winkler's intestinal tract, plus a huge tapeworm 11 feet long.

Mrs. Winkler also expelled worms with every enema until March 17, 1958. However, neither of them were able to completely conquer the worms until they went on a raw papaya diet, with nothing but papaya for six days, then juices for six days, followed by another six days on papaya. That, thank goodness, was the *end* of the worm problem!

Regarding the enemas and colonics, Winkler writes, "We were taught before coming to the Kay-El-Bar Ranch that colonics and enemas were *dangerous.* Now I can truthfully say that they have saved our lives and brought abundant health to both of us!"

Before leaving Wickenburg, Frank and Emma Jean Winkler decided to go "all the way" in the program of

healthful living, as taught by Dr. Walker. They detei-
mined that henceforth they would eat nothing but raw
fruits and vegetables and the juices from these live foods.
It was a pretty big decision for these two former gourmets
to make. But their decision was final and irrevocable.

On returning home, without so much as a parting tear,
the Winklers tossed out their beautiful electric range, and
in its place, they lovingly installed the gleaming new
juicer. With almost religious zeal, they next cleaned
out the medicine cabinet — containing almost a bushel-
basketful of drugs, potions and pills — and threw
them into the ash can. Then they called in their neighbors and friends and gave away all their flour, sugar,
canned goods and processed foodstuffs until the cup-
boards were bare!

For three years now, this enlightened family has not
touched a mouthful of cooked or processed food. No
meat, no fish or fowl, no eggs, no milk, cream or cheese —
no canned goods of any description, and no legumes have
appeared on their still bountiful table. What is the
result or fruitage of all this "sacrifice" of the *culinary
arts* in this home? For an answer let's listen to Frank
Winkler's own personal testimony:

"Without surgery and without drug medication of
any kind — *gone* is the bothersome *constipation! Gone*
are the painful bleeding *hemorrhoids!* Gone are the
noxious devitalizing *worms! Gone* is all that superfluous
fat! And *gone* forever, thank God, is the grim spectre
of *death* that haunted me for so long following the
doctor's frightening prognosis. While the bladder tumors
have not entirely disappeared as yet, they apparently have
been brought under control, and no longer constitute a
'Sword of Damocles' hanging over my head and threaten-
ing to terminate my earthly career.

"At the age of 62, my weight is precisely what it
should be — not one pound *over* nor one pound *under* —
but just right for my height (5 feet 8 inches), an even

156 pounds! At long last I have experienced the joy of *eating to live!* — not just living to eat!"

Are you ill — suffering from some so-called "incurable malady?" If so, it might be well for you to consider the example set for these two doughty pioneers in diet reform.

During their first visit on Sunday afternoon, January 10, 1960, at my Monrovia home, Frank and Emma Jean Winkler not only related their interesting case histories, but they also gave me their daily menu — the most important single factor, not only in their remarkable recovery, but in their present state of vibrant good health. This menu is of such value that I wish to pass it on to my readers for their study and edification.

As a physician interested in the healing and restorative power of nature, I wish to commend this simple diet to all my friends who may be suffering from distressing chronic ailments and the all-too-prevalent diseases of physical degeneration.

This program, by the way, is nothing *new*. In fact raw fruits and vegetables, just as they came from the hand of the Creator, were among the foods given to man in the Garden of Eden. And according to the Scriptural record, those hardy primeval ancestors of ours lived to the almost incredible age of 1,000 years! So, if the Winkler program is "faddism" — let's have more of the same! At least they are in "tune" with the Creator!

Listen, while the Winklers tell in their own words the details of their "new way of life."

"First thing in the morning we take the juice of one lemon in warm water. One-half hour after the drink, we eat our breakfast of whatever fresh fruit is available. This winter we have been eating grapefruit for breakfast — organically-grown grapefruit whenever possible.

"During the middle of the morning we each drink a pint of carrot juice. At noon our meal consists of a huge vegetable salad weighing from three to four pounds. Often there are up to seventeen different kinds of vegetables in this salad. Of course this salad is made for two persons. We use no nuts or fruits of any kind with these vegetable salads. As a dressing we use lemon juice, safflower oil and honey seasoning it with a vegetable seasoning, alfalfa, sweet basil, kelp, tahini, etc. The dressing is made with our blender. We change the *base* each day for the sake of variety.

"About 1:30 in the afternoon we take a pint of carrot juice each, and at 3:30 a second pint of the same. For supper we eat whatever fruit is available in season — persimmons, apples, grapes, pears, nectarines, or papaya, which is our favorite fruit; but we never mix two kinds of fruits at the same meal. We eat about two pounds of fruit apiece for supper.

"At 7:30 in the evening we each take another pint of carrot juice. Freshly pressed fruit juices are sometimes substituted. We often mix the juices from green leaves in with the carrot juice. These include such potent juices as parsley, celery, watercress, dandelion, kale, etc.

"We have found by long experience this menu supplies *all* our dietetic requirements including the important protein factor, and keeps us both in a state of good health the year around."

Today this happy, vibrant-with-life couple live five months of each year in the trailer they purchased in 1957. They love to travel and enjoy good, organically-grown foods so abundant now in Southern California. By the way, the most important piece of equipment in the Winkler Mobile Home is their precious juicer. It travels with them whenever and wherever they go.

In bringing this chapter to a close, I cannot help but agree with the Winklers, who in turn follow the teachings of Hippocrates, Father of Medicine, when he declared: "Leave your drugs in the chemist's pot if you can heal the patient with *food.*"

CHAPTER FOURTEEN

CAN I NOT ENJOY THE FOOD I LIKE AND BE HEALTHY? CERTAINLY, IF YOU FIRST MAKE SURE YOU GET THE FOOD YOU NEED. SCIENTISTS IN THE FIELD OF NUTRITION SEEM TO BE UNANIMOUS IN AGREEING THAT ONE-HALF OF ALL CALORIES SHOULD COME FROM RAW VEGETABLES, FRUITS AND MILK PRODUCTS.

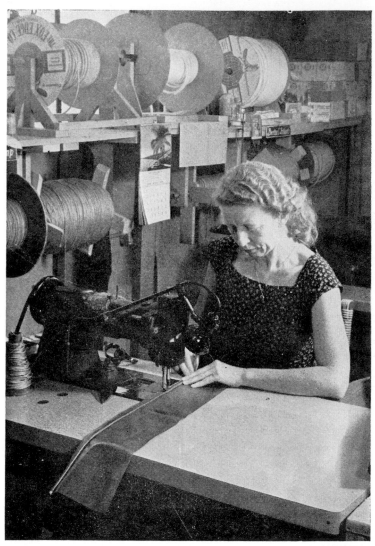

Mrs. A. the once hopeless arthritic, now works hard all day in a large upholstering plant in Monrovia. Here she is at one of the many large sewing machines. She takes a half-gallon jug of carrot juice with her to the shop each day. For her thrilling story turn to page 51. After her busy day at the factory she says: "I could dance all night!" Here indeed is a "modern miracle"!

The Voice of
Experience

M Y FIRST heart attack was in February, 1942. I spent
eight weeks in the St. Helena Sanitarium and Hospital. I was unable to walk for the following three or four
weeks. I suffered pain and attacks which kept me at home
for the next eight or nine months. I started work on my
old job after a year's absence; but as soon as I would work
a little too hard, back to the hospital I would go.

"Then in 1948, to aggravate my condition, I was
afflicted with arthritis. This condition became steadily
worse. I spent hundreds of dollars on doctors and pre-
scriptions. Two fingers on my left hand were crippled.
In 1953, neuritis and bursitis set in my back, shoulders
and arms; also my right leg and hip, which left me in
terrible pain. I was now completely helpless.

"I took hypos and drugs until I got my juicer in
October, 1953. I drank from two to three quarts of carrot
and celery juice daily. In nine weeks, all my pain had
left. In less than a year, my fingers which were stiff,
straightened up so that I could use them again.

"I also had prostate gland trouble for over seven
years. I had to go to the bathroom from six to seven
times at night. I went to the doctor's every Thursday
for a massage and treatment, without any relief, which
took a lot of time and money. Since taking my juices,
I have positively cured my prostate gland condition. I
would take two ounces of pure parsley juice from three
to four times daily.

"In fact, I have no arthritis or neuritis or prostate
gland trouble since, and my heart is getting stronger
rapidly."

LETTER NUMBER TWO

"Previous to my having access to the juice, I was forced to be faithful to a rigid diet of goat milk and soft boiled eggs. It was an extremely difficult situation trying to perform a day's labor on such a diet. After receiving the advice of a number of people and the good news contained in a book, recommended by you, confirming the fact that the raw vegetable juices would help relieve my ulcerous stomach condition, I purchased a machine. I can gratefully say the cabbage, celery, and carrot juices proved their healing power in my case. Even though my stomach no longer bothers me, I am continuing to drink the juice. In fact, my wife and I consider the juices the most refreshing and nourishing beverage one can consume any time of the day or night."

LETTER NUMBER THREE

"I am sixty-seven, and the arthritis does not bother me any more. I went to a doctor for many months, tried eliminating certain foods, took different kinds of medicine; had short wave treatments, and gold shots, etc., and still got worse instead of better. Prior to taking treatments from this doctor, I had tried two different kinds of vitamin courses, that cost more than the juicer did, and still did not get results.

"I was getting to be rather helpless, as it hurt to wring out my wash cloth, lift a dish, or do any housework. I was constantly rubbing my hands when I could, to try and relieve the hurt; knitted a lot to try and keep my hands supple. I was about to sell my automobile, as it hurt so to drive, or hold the wheel. It even hurt to pull the bed covers over me; and it was commencing to hurt in different parts of my body. I visualized myself as a helpless cripple. Then — we bought the juice extractor, and that was May 14, 1949. I used the juices as recommended, with the result that one day about three months later.

I realized I was without a pain, or any discomfort. I had not kept track and so how much sooner I was healed, I do not know, but it definitely was done. And now at this writing I am still entirely well, and of course keep on using the juices. It is wonderful to be able to again be active with no hurt to pain, or discomfort."

LETTER NUMBER FOUR

During the cherry harvest of 1949 I began to go down hill very rapidly. I had to force myself to keep going. For several years I had realized that something was seriously wrong, but would not give up, and continued to "carry on." After cherry harvest, however, I went to see Dr B, who was highly recommended to me. After a thorough examination he informed me that the mouth of my bladder had grown shut, and that I would have to undergo surgery. On October 2nd, 1949 I entered Community Hospital and was operated on. The surgeon removed a cancer.

Before I got out of the hospital I developed a blood clot in both legs, and was compelled to remain for another two months. After coming home I made no improvement, and a short while later a blood clot also developed in my lungs. I was taken to a nearby Sanitarium for treatment. After returning home, my heart was so bad I couldn't walk across the street without collapsing, and for two years I sat with my feet propped up. My old "ticker" didn't have enough power to pump the blood either to my feet or my head. The doctors told me that I might possibly live a year if I kept quiet — but no more.

Then I found some literature on the therapeutic value of live food juices. The idea appealed to me. I was desperate and willing to try anything. I figured I had nothing to lose and possibly something to gain. So I bought a juicer and commenced to drink quantities of carrot and celery juice — within a month up to one-half gallon a day

I immediately began to gain — and after four years I am still at it — using one quart of the juices every day.

LETTER NUMBER FIVE

"I am writing you about the vegetable juices and what they have done for our family. Since February, 1956 we have used lots of celery, spinach, carrot and parsley juices. My father-in-law has been afflicted with diabetes for twenty years, and was taking 15 units of Insulin. On February 28th, 1956, after only twenty days on the live food juices he was taking five units, and was eating many more things than he had ever been able to do. He feels better and looks better, and he is seventy-nine years old! What is more he is active and works every day. We are all thrilled about the vegetable and fruit juices, and think they are wonderful."

———◇———

Dr. Bircher-Benner Recommends LIVE FOOD JUICES

"Juices are far superior to a milk diet. They are invaluable against diseases of metabolism such as gout and obesity. What is aimed at in such cases is the temporary reduction of food to a minimum in order to obtain the combustion of fat, to neutralize the poisoning effects of uric acid and to bring about its excretion. Anyone who understands how to observe such cases will be convinced of the astonishing nutritive power of this food. These nutritive juices are as it were, the 'mother's milk' of those who are seriously ill, the only food they are still able to take. But they are not to be considered as mere beverages. The patient is not to *drink* them, he is to *eat* them. One small spoonful after another is to be taken and slowly swallowed." — Dr. M. Bircher-Benner.

CHAPTER FIFTEEN

"IN CASE OF SICKNESS, THE CAUSE
SHOULD BE ASCERTAINED, UN-
HEALTHFUL CONDITIONS SHOULD
BE CHANGED, WRONG HABITS
CORRECTED. THEN NATURE IS TO
BE ASSISTED IN HER EFFORT TO
EXPEL IMPURITIES AND TO RE-
ESTABLISH RIGHT CONDITIONS IN
THE SYSTEM."

— Ministry of Healing, page 127.

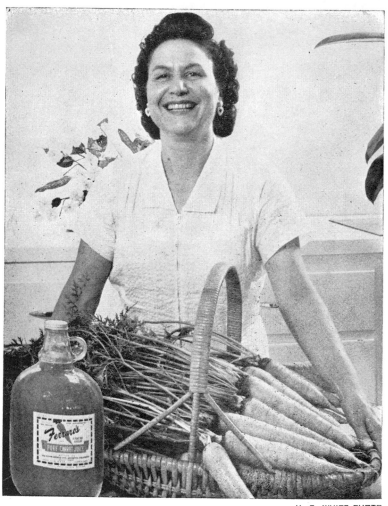

Believe it or not this radiant personality is none other than our famous "Mrs. X." She attributes her miraculous restoration to a diet of one gallon of carrot juice per day over a period of eighteen months. Her splendid health and tireless energy are maintained on a low protein diet consisting of carrot juice only during the day, and in the evening, a large raw vegetable salad, avocado, sunflower and sesame seeds, and a few nuts. This recent picture is proof positive of the miraculous power of simple, raw juices to re-build a sick, starving body to a condition of **optimal health.** (See illustration on page 30.)

This Question
of Protein

ONE OF THE MOST frequent questions asked about the raw juice diet is: "Where will I obtain the proteins that my body needs?" When I refer my questioners to the experience of Mrs. X (the carrot-juice woman), it is difficult for them to believe that anyone could gain seventy pounds in eighteen months on a diet of carrot juice alone — with no other supplementary sources of protein.

The remarkable restoration of Mrs. X took place ten years ago, and since then fresh raw juices with a salad each day have been this busy woman's diet. Her radiant personality and vibrant good health are reflected in the accompanying photograph taken only a few months ago. (See frontispiece.) For Mrs. X the controversial "Protein Question" has been forever settled. She finds adequate protein of the highest nutritional quality in a simple diet of raw juices and leafy vegetables!

But, what about the high protein diet thought now to be so essential as to require the use of flesh foods? For an authoritative answer to this important question, let me refer my readers to some of the world's leading research scientists in the field of nutrition. Their experiments, observation, and mature conclusion may prove helpful to those of us who want to KNOW the truth.

Dr. L. H. Newburgh, of the University of Michigan, Ann Arbor, is regarded as one of America's leading physiological chemists. In rat feeding experiments, this scientist started with 15% protein, which was a normal rat diet. He then added meat protein up to 25%. According to the record, "the rats showed bigger growth and more activity than normal controls, but in one and one-half

111

years their kidneys showed advanced Bright's Disease. The appearance of the rats," declared Dr. Newburgh, "was no index of what was taking place in their kidneys." As he pushed the meat diet higher (up to 80% of their food) the kidney damage appeared earlier and was more severe. At the conclusion of his experiments he observed: "Protein is awfully poor fuel for heat and energy" — too much SLAG!

In a book "The Nutrition of Man," the distinguished physiological chemist, Dr. Russell Chittenden of Yale University, calls attention to the fact that the American diet is far too high in protein, and especially meat protein. This noted scientist proved conclusively that not only could the daily amount of protein be *reduced* to as low as 50 grams or less, but also proved that such a "lowering of the protein greatly increased the health, endurance, and working power of the individual."

Some time ago Owen S. Parrett, M.D., long-time researcher and advocate of a low protein diet, wrote to Dr. Frederick J. Stare, head of the department of Nutrition, Harvard School of Public Health. This leader in the field of nutrition answered Dr. Parrett's questions as follows:

1. Question: Is meat essential to an adequate diet?
   Answer: "It is possible to have an adequate diet without consuming meat."
2. Question: What is your standard requirement of protein per day?
   Answer: "It is desirable to consume somewhere between 60 and 100 grams of protein per day. With adequate calories in the diet the amount of protein for an adult can probably be reduced to as low as 40 grams."
3. Question: Do whole grain cereals furnish complete proteins?
   Answer: "Cereals are good sources of protein and when used in the proper mixture will supply *complete protein.*"

4. Question: Can an adequate diet be secured without meat, eggs, or milk?

 Answer: "It is not absolutely necessary that milk and eggs be included in the diet if meat is omitted; as *adequate protein* can be obtained by using mixed whole grains, legumes and nuts."

In his thesis on "PROTEINS," Lloyd K. Rosenvold, M.D., of Montrose, Colorado, agrees with Drs. Newburgh, Chittenden, and Stare. He states that "A few years ago it was thought that a high protein diet (100-150 grams per day) was essential. Recent information, however, seems to indicate that if *good quality* protein is used the total amount need not be so great. . . . Vegetarians, though sometimes impaired in efficiency, thrive on 40 60 grams of protein at 70 Kilograms body weight. A case illustrative of this was a physician, aged 48, who maintained normal physical ability and normal chemical composition of the blood on a daily caloric intake of 1600-1800 calories, and a daily protein intake of only 30-40 grams. His only source of animal protein was 80 cc. of milk daily."

"Another physician, Dr. C. Rose, lived for fifteen years with a daily intake of 38-40 grams of protein, and during this period, without signs of unusual fatigue or exhaustion, climbed twenty-two mountain peaks, including the formidable Matterhorn."

From the *American Journal of Public Health,* I present a report from Dr. Frederick J. Stare and George W. Thorn as follows: "Interesting data on dietary protein and signs of protein deficiency have recently been reported by Youmans. Out of a group of approximately 1,100 individuals in Tennessee that were studied in considerable detail, there were some 40% who had a dietary protein intake of less than 50 grams daily. In these 450 individuals who had been receiving less than 50 grams of protein per day, probably for most of their lives, only 5 subjects or less than 1% had clinical evidence of protein deficiency.

Furthermore, the caloric intake of these individuals was in general low, and it is entirely possible that with an adequate caloric intake no signs of protein deficiency would have occurred."

All this scientific testimony from leading authorities in the field of nutrition takes on added weight when we realize that we are here dealing with the most important factor in the composition of our bodies. Protein has been called "the essence of life," and in a very real sense, that is true of all animal and vegetable life. Proteins are the "building blocks" out of which the structure of physical existence is composed. It is to the human what steel is to the automobile; and it wears out just as steel wears out, and must be replaced through our food.

There are many forms of proteins, and we have heard much emphasis to the effect that animal protein is the most important. But this is not necessarily true. I have in my hand at the present moment a book in which there has been collaboration by six leading authorities in the medical and bio-chemistry fields, and here is a direct statement made by them:

"Whether proteins in the food are of animal or plant origin is completely immaterial, since they are all broken down into their amino acids before they can be built into the structure of the body; as no protein molecule in the condition in which it exists either in plant or animal can be absorbed into the bloodstream until it is broken down into its component amino acids."

Dr. Sherman, eminent nutritional authority of Columbia University states that the energy needs of the body can be far better met by carbohydrates than by protein. Furthermore, if we follow what Dr. Sherman points out, that one-half the calories taken as food should be in the form of vegetables and fruits, our nutritional needs will be adequately taken care of. We will have no need to fear a protein deficiency.

CHAPTER SIXTEEN

"AGRICULTURAL AND NUTRI-
TIONAL SCIENCE CAN BANISH BOTH
HUNGER AND MALNUTRITION
FROM THE EXPERIENCE OF OUR
PEOPLE ALMOST AS COMPLETELY
AS BACTERIAL SCIENCE BANISHED
YELLOW FEVER AND CHOLERA...."

— *N. Philip Norman, M.D.*

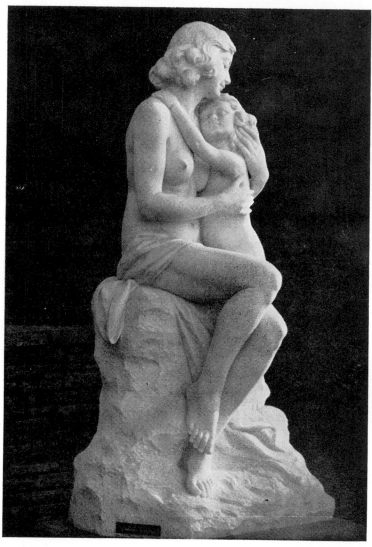

H. C. WHITE PHOTO

This enchanting photograph of one of Forest Lawn's most beautiful statues, is a fitting symbol of woman's grace, tenderness and beauty. Every line of this lovely figure in marble reveals the role of "correct nutrition" in building "The Body Beautiful."

The Body Beautiful
By Movie Actress Ingeborg Loff

YOU'VE seen me on magazine covers and in pictures. But I want you to know at twenty-five no one living would have wanted my picture.

"My figure was dumpy, my complexion like the bottom of a dried river. I had little watery eyes and no eyelashes. My hair was a matted mass of colorless twine. My few acquaintances called me dull, stupid, and even a natural born idiot. The only thing that really interested me was sleeping. No man ever asked twice to take me out. I had been to a splendid school. My father and mother were wonderful people, but I had all the appearances of a scrub-woman of fifty when I was only twenty-five. I couldn't secure work of a mental order. In terrible discouragement I applied for a housekeeping position. It was with a Scandinavian doctor in New York City.

"After I had worked for him a week he asked me if he could experiment with me promising that nothing would hurt me, that I was a chemical plant like everything else in Nature, and that if I would let him make me over, he would see that I was helped to the top in better ways.

"It required a week of experimental work on his part before I realized that I was beginning to think and look differently. It seemed strange. He fed me special meals six times a day. I had no white bread or starch of any kind. He made me drink small drinks of vegetable juices several times daily. Once a week I was shown before a group of doctors who were studying bio-chemistry with the doctor. They all took notes on my change in hair, color of eyes, depth of chest, greater slenderness of ankles, and they pinched my skin to note how it changed each week. I was getting a marvelous complexion. My hair was glowing, and was turning lighter with golden tints in it. I wanted to run and shout for the sheer joy of living. My finger nails, my eyebrows and lashes were growing better and developing a gloss. The fat lumps about my hips had disappeared. I lost twenty-five pounds and yet I had been eating oftener. I became fired with ambition. My mind and heart went out to new studies, new people, and I know I had never really lived before I had been analyzed by this doctor."

— From *The Body Beautiful,* an American Magazine.

Formula for Dr. Kirschner's Therapeutic

GREEN DRINK

15 Almonds   4 Pitted Dates
5 Teaspoonfuls Sunflower Seeds
(Soak overnight in water)

Fill the liquifier above the blades with unsweetened pineapple juice. (Approximately 8 ounces). Place the softened nuts, seeds and dates in the pineapple juice and liquify. Pour this mixture into a pitcher.

Next, take four large handfuls of green leaves — such as alfalfa, parsley, mint, spinach, beet greens, water-cress; and if obtainable, comfrey and such nutritious weeds as fillaree, malva, or lambs' quarters. (Do not use stems.)

Liquify the greens in 8 ounces of unsweetened pineapple juice. Then put the two mixtures together and stir.

Caution: Do not have the mixture too thick. Some like to put the combined mixture through a coarse sieve or strainer before serving to eliminate the pulp.

MUSELI

(The Delicious Raw Porridge Formulated by the late
Dr. Bircher-Benner)

The portion for one person is as follows:

(1) 2 small apples, or one large apple
(2) 1 tablespoonful almonds, walnuts,
   pecans or hazel-nuts (grated)
(3) 1 tablespoonful rolled oats — previously
   soaked for 12 hours in water
(4) Juice of half a lemon
(5) 1 tablespoon of top milk or cream
(6) Honey to taste.

First mix the cream and honey and lemon juice with
the rolled oats. Then grate the apple — including the skin,
core and seeds — into the mixture with a two-way grater.
Stir continuously. The grated nuts are then sprinkled
over the dish to increase protein and fat values.

OTHER BOOKS ON RELATED TOPICS

Those of my readers who have been helped by the
message of hope contained in this little volume will also
be interested in my other two books — NATURE'S
HEALING GRASSES and ARE YOU WHAT YOU
EAT? More than 100,000 copies of these "Help-Yourself-
to-Better-Health" books have been sold in four years.

Here is what other medical doctors have to say about
these books: "You have reduced scientific findings into a
workable, understandable text . . . Capable of holding the
interest of the most skeptical." "The story you are trying
to get over to the public is PREVENTION. It is the
basis of the therapy for the coming generation."

Postscript . . .

IN CONCLUDING our treatise on the therapeutic value of live food juices, I wish to make it plain that it is quite impossible within the scope of a single book to give more than a brief glimpse into this challenging phase of dietetics and its growing influence in the field of curative and preventive medicine.

In LIVE FOOD JUICES I have endeavored to portray to you some of the exciting possibilities in store for *you* through the use of these natural life-giving and life-sustaining FOODS. If it has helped you to discover some new sources of LIFE and HEALTH this book will have fulfilled the purpose of the author.

In conclusion I wish to express my deep appreciation to all those who have assisted in the preparation of this volume:

To Dr. Fred D. Miller for his splendid Introduction.

To Kay K. Thomas, Editor of *Let's Live,* and Herbert C. White, for their invaluable editorial assistance.

To the U. S. Department of Agriculture, the Universities and Research Centers, who have so generously contributed their technical knowledge in preparing the chapters on Mineral and Vitamin Sources.

To the publishers of *The Body Beautiful* for the inspiring story of Movie Actress Ingeborg Loff.

To the Union Pacific Railway, the U. S. Department of Agriculture, and Photographer Herbert Clarence White, for the use of their splendid photographs.

To one and all of you — My HEARTFELT THANKS! — The Author.